Praise for He

"Micah has created a must-read for anyone cu... power of psychedelics. *Healing Psychedelics* demystifies the process and emphasizes safety and effectiveness, making it an essential guide for both new explorers and seasoned practitioners to dive deeper into the world of psychedelics. Read this book and discover how psychedelics can transform your journey through trauma."

—**Jessika Lagarde, psychedelic-assisted medicine facilitator, integration coach, and cofounder of Women On Psychedelics**

"Micah's book finally gives us and the world of psychedelics a book that does justice to the long and often lengthy process of using psychedelics to support healing trauma. Her honest description of this process highlights both challenges and the great rewards that lie ahead of anyone seeking to use psychedelics for healing their trauma. As a seasoned psychedelic therapist myself, I am relieved that Micah has written this book as it brings attention to the not-so-quick-fix nature of these experiences, sheds light on the cultural narrative of the 'panacea' that surrounds psychedelic medicine, and brings the reader a more realistic view of the healing journey these medicine journeys are here to carry us through."

—**Dori G. Lewis she/her, MA, EdM, LPC-S, co-owner and cofounder of *elementalpsychedelics.com***

"Micah bravely addresses both the light and shadow encountered when a therapist and client embark on this transformative journey together. She touches on the origins of this medicine honoring indigenous teachers who have protected and shared it for centuries. Through her expertise and compassionate insight, Micah illustrates how a carefully nurtured therapeutic relationship has the potential to change not just individuals, but the world."

—**Rev. Liliana Barzola, curandera and founder of Lotus Lantern Healing Arts**

Healing Psychedelics

INNOVATIVE THERAPIES FOR TRAUMA AND TRANSFORMATION

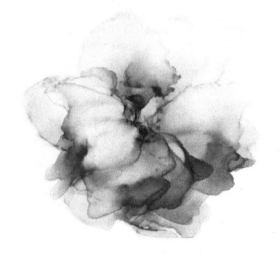

MICAH STOVER

FOREWORD BY CRAIG HEACOCK, MD

HAMPTON ROADS

This edition first published in 2024 by Hampton Roads Publishing, an imprint of

Red Wheel/Weiser, LLC
With offices at:
65 Parker Street, Suite 7
Newburyport, MA 01950

Sign up for our newsletter and special offers
by going to *www.redwheelweiser.com/newsletter*

Cover design by Brittany Craig
Cover and interior image by iStock
Interior by Steve Amarillo / Urban Design LLC
Typeset in Minion Pro, Montserrat, and Gill Sans

ISBN: 978-1-64297-064-7
Names: Stover, Micah, 1979- author.
Title: Healing psychedelics : innovative therapies for trauma and
transformation / Micah Stover ; foreword Craig Heacock.
Description: Newburyport, MA : Hampton Roads Publishing, [2024] | Includes
bibliographical references and index. | Summary: "Psychedelics are
showing great promise as a new way to heal trauma and improve emotional
wellness. This book offers a comprehensive and informative guide for
both professionals and patients who are interested in learning more
about psychedelic-assisted therapy"-- Provided by publisher.
Identifiers: LCCN 2024007434 | ISBN 9781642970647 | ISBN 9781612835037
(ebook)
Subjects: LCSH: Hallucinogenic drugs. | Post-traumatic stress
disorder--Treatment. | BISAC: BODY, MIND & SPIRIT / Entheogens &
Visionary Substances | SOCIAL SCIENCE / Popular Culture
Classification: LCC BF209.H34 S76 2024 | DDC 154.4--dc23/eng/20240809
LC record available at https://lccn.loc.gov/2

Printed in the United States of America
IBI
10 9 8 7 6 5 4 3 2 1

Dedication

May these stories and the vulnerability reflected through them be an eternal offering to:

My children for breaking my heart out of the bottle,

My partner for loving me through the mess,

My ancestors for the epigenetic material required to create my life,

My village for their nurture and support,

My clients for the gift of being their witness.

Contents

Foreword

PSYCHEDELIC MEDICINES DO THEIR MAGIC in at least four major realms—the brain, the mind, the spirit, and the interpersonal/transferential space. Much has been written of how psychedelics change the brain, plumb the psyche, and connect us to the greater anima/spirit. And while these explanations are all central to understanding how psychedelics "work," what is too often ignored is arguably the most powerful force in the room—that of the connection between client/patient/journeyer and therapist/guide (from now on I'll use "therapist" and "client" as a proxy for these various roles).

At the heart of therapy is the therapist-client dynamic, and more specifically how the client inevitably begins to experience the therapist through the experiential lens of a child in the presence of a critical and all-powerful adult—often a parent or primary caregiver. Therapists take on unique powers in their role as the holders of this relationship, allowing their clients to work through wounds and traumas that live on and continue to shape their selves and their experience of the world.

Psychedelics can open the heart, connecting us to the loving energy that fills us and binds us to everyone and everything. By cranking up love and trust, they turn up the transference dial to 11, allowing for an even more rapid and profound exploration of early childhood dynamics and trauma. Transference, as a key element of psychedelic therapy, has as much healing potential as does the psychedelic medicine itself. This is because most early childhood trauma is related to an absence of safe connection and/or a presence of threat.

As a therapist in the psychedelic space, we embody the placeholder of mother and father, of feminine and masculine. This provides an opportunity for clients to cast the pain of the past onto a fresh canvas, and in so doing, gain the potential for a corrective experience. Therapists can provide the safety and validation clients lacked in childhood, and, when that happens, individuals have the opportunity to reconsolidate their sense of self. Alternatively, psychedelics can spark a compelling romantic transference, convincing clients and/or therapists that they are falling in love. This supercharging of the transference can lead to unintentional and unconscious boundary crossings and violations, including inappropriate touch and even sexual transgressions.

Anyone working in the psychedelic space must come to understand and respect the power of psychedelic-augmented transference and its potential outcomes. We can use these medicines to deepen the therapeutic relationship and thus the course of healing, or we can ignore this reality at our peril.

I'm so honored that Micah asked me to write this foreword. All of you readers are in for such a treat. Micah comes to this space with so much experience and wisdom and compassion and humility. I think she's the perfect person to introduce you to the therapeutic possibilities of the psychedelic realm, especially the power and healing inherent in the therapeutic relationship.

Craig Heacock, MD
Host of Back from the Abyss *podcast*

Introduction:
History and Context
of Psychedelics

THE HISTORY OF WORKING WITH AND USING PSYCHEDELICS is deep and complex, ranging from ancient indigenous practices to a more volatile past in the archives of American culture. The 1960s and 1970s are stored in our collective memory as the first "psychedelic renaissance"—a time of Vietnam War protests and the counter-capitalist uprising of the Woodstock era. They were a time in which people like Timothy Leary rocked the status quo with famous sentiments like: "Turn on, tune in, drop out."

This is where our minds go when we think of psychedelics. This liberal counter-culture movement, in which psychedelics like psilocybin and LSD played a significant role, followed by a firm, patriarchal reaction known as "the war on drugs," in which Richard Nixon and Ronald Reagan after him squelched ongoing research and discoveries that focused on how psychedelic medicines could support people in states of despair and crisis. This escalated beyond the defunding of research and made the use and consumption of these medicines the scapegoat for emerging problems in American culture that were summarized with one scary word: *crime.*

Opponents to this reactionary response, like Terence McKenna, became famous with statements like: "Psychedelics are illegal not because a loving government is concerned that you may jump out of a third-story window

. . . [but because] they open you up to the possibility that everything you know is wrong." The war on drugs marked a temporary and unfortunate pause in one of the most important mental-health conversations of our time—and, dare I say, our humanity. And this is true even without getting into the implicit and explicit socio-political and racial implications that persist today in the backlash of this war.

Fast forward fifty or sixty years. In some ways, we have come full circle. We've cycled back to reopening this dialog and unearthing the research. Only now, we've added critical layers. The recent global pandemic brought the world to its knees and forced us to reckon with the gravity and pervasiveness of the mental-health crisis in ways we'd been desperately trying to manage and avoid. In 2004, the Multidisciplinary Association for Psychedelic Studies (MAPS) began clinical trials for patients suffering from PTSD (post-traumatic stress syndrome) and CPTSD (complex post-traumatic stress syndrome), leveraging drugs like MDMA as a psychedelic tool to help facilitate a process of healing and recovery.

MDMA, in street verbiage, is often referred to as "ecstacy." But it is important to note here that medical-grade MDMA and ecstacy are not necessarily the same thing. MDMA at medical grade is a pure compound, while ecstacy is typically less pure.

The outcomes of these clinical trials were jaw-droppingly positive. Although the shadow of the war on drugs still looms large, the data that emerged from these studies spoke directly to the urgency of the problem and the desperation to find new solutions. And this marked the beginning of our current psychedelic renaissance.

To my surprise and initial resistance, I found myself in the middle of this new movement, this *uprising*, as a patient. I was a person in crisis, desperate to heal. Following a traumatic birth, in which both my son and I nearly died, I faced a reservoir of unearthed complex trauma and knew I needed to be better for myself and for my son—a need that I now understand as a landslide of epigenetic and intergenerational trauma that required far more than talk therapy to repair.

Today, I am a certified psychedelic-assisted somatic therapist who has spent hundreds of hours at the side of innumerable clients navigating this process of healing. I've trained with some of the best in the field and I have become an advocate who works with reverence, commitment, and intention to promote education and awareness of how this therapy can safely bring about optimal outcomes.

We stand today on the brink of great possibility—or the precipice of disaster. Does that sound dramatic? It is. The health of our future depends, at least in part, on this conversation. This is what makes transparency and an expanding archive of real resources so critical to where we are now. The holistic health of our collective future as a people and a planet depends on this roll of the dice. How we move forward, given the gravity of what's at stake, will ultimately determine the extent to which these extraordinary medicinal tools will be part of the solution.

If you think the stakes sound high, they are. With deep reverence, from a grounded place, I say that the risks of not pivoting now are grave. Consider a relatively small sample of recent statistics. During the recent pandemic, the World Health Organization reported a 25 percent increase in the prevalence of anxiety and depression.[1] Boston University School of Public Health published an article citing that the rates of depression within the United States had tripled, suggesting that *one in three Americans* suffer with depression and/or anxiety.[2]

If that's not enough, consider how these trends are directly impacting women, children, and the American family. Five hundred thousand people in the US experience sexual assault or abuse each year and 60,000 of those are children. More than 4.5 million people received treatment at a specialty facility or mental-health service in the past year. According to the American Association for Marriage and Family Therapy, 1.8 million people are in therapy, served by 55,000 therapists.[3] These numbers are just a small sample from a larger pool of emerging data that continues to make headlines weekly, illuminating the scope and impact of our current mental-health crisis.

This is not to suggest that, if we all start consuming psychedelics, our problems will be solved and our planet saved. That would be painfully naive and grossly reductionist. But it is to intentionally state that hurt people . . . hurt people. We are living in a time when far more people are hurting than thriving. That must change. While these problems are multi-layered and many things are needed to facilitate that change, I firmly believe that psychedelics are critical to the solution. Moreover, many others agree. Look at the radical success of Michael Pollan's ground-breaking book, now a television docu-series, *How to Change Your Mind*, as well as many others. Central to all these efforts is a conviction that mental-health issues and the possibility of increased healing intersect with a discussion of psychedelics.

We don't have to look very hard or very far to see the proliferation of content in traditional and social media that is focused on these cultural concerns of imbalance and dysfunction—and the potential for psychedelics to be part of the healing and recovery toolbox. Within the last three years, the *New York Times*, for example, has repeatedly run articles with headlines like: "A Psychedelic Drug Passes a Big Test for PTSD Treatment."[4] Several dozen podcasts focused on psychedelic-assisted therapy are already available online. Conferences like Psychedelic Science 2023, hosted by MAPS, are drawing thousands of researchers, activists, and practitioners from countries around the world.

The potential for this renewed discussion rests on our capacity to learn from the past and to increase transparency and conversation without secrets or shame. We must use the wealth of available research and data, as well as advances in science that address how psychedelics can work for us.

A Leap of Faith

When my family moved to Mexico from Portland, Oregon, I was immersed in the underground psychedelic community and on my clinical path of study and training. Even undertaking the move to a foreign country, to sell all our possessions, felt "psychedelic" and reflected the internal changes brought about by my own healing journey. Prior to experiencing psychedelic therapy, it would have been inconceivable for me to take a leap that bold without a perfectly clear plan. The idea of moving and beginning anew with our small children in a more affordable place where we hoped to achieve a greater semblance of work-life balance felt more romantic in theory than the actual experience of landing in a totally different culture with no support community, only a limited ability to speak the language, and not a clue of how to find resources we were accustomed to having at our fingertips in the United States.

In the absence of conveniences like next-day package delivery and the buffet of organic foods and supplements I'd grown accustomed to, I felt stripped of security and a familiar sense of panic re-emerged. I found myself questioning everything I'd felt confident about only three weeks before as we embarked on the great family adventure of our lives. I felt foolish, scared, and irresponsible, and wondered how I was going to take care of my kids and myself in this place where everything flowed so differently.

As is true for many who become "cycle-breakers" in an intergenerational line of traumatic wounds and dysfunction, I realized that space and boundaries can help greatly to shift perspective and hold safety in situations that initially feel impossible to navigate. Space doesn't have to mean moving to a foreign country, but it does require new internal and external boundaries and beliefs relating to the people and things that activate our nervous system.

For me, moving to Mexico felt like molting, like a snake slithering out of an old skin that no longer fit its body. Adapting to the much slower, nonurgent pace of life in Mexico was at once a salve to my nervous system and entirely activating. I was dying to slow down, but at the same time I felt lost as to what to do when I tried to sit still.

The Earth As Mother

As the days, weeks, and months passed, we built what I now refer to with clients as our "village of care." Many of the local practitioners and *curanderos/ curanderas* I met worked with indigenous medicines and practices. With their guidance, I came to recognize that, beyond training and professional certifications and degrees—what stood out as distinct from everything and everyone I'd worked with in the US—was how their cultural ethos included solid connection to community, to nature, and to the Earth itself. And that is when the experience of Earth as Mother began to solidify for me. I repeatedly heard some version of this same message: *Secure attachment begins with your connection to the Earth.* While the notion of Mother Nature was not new to me, my experience of her as alive, communicative, and relationally engaged was categorically different.

As I studied the indigenous ways of relating to the Earth and the Earth's medicines, like psilocybin, I started to hear and experience the medicine as a conduit for tuning into the Earth Mother's wisdom and voice. I noticed how the people around me had some sort of intimate relationship with a vast maternal presence referred to as *Pachamama,* a name that had roots in Incan traditions and indigenous people of the Andes. Pachamama was believed to be an eternal loving presence who governed fertility, the harvest, and natural cycles like the seasons, as well as storms, earthquakes, and floods. The relationship to Pachamama was integral to abundance in life. She was the great giver. Honoring her generosity required cultivating a spirit of reciprocity within ourselves. In other words, we must learn to give as much—if not more—than we take. Throughout the chapters and stories that follow, you will hear and experience the voice of Pachamama as she was introduced to me. You will gain a sense of how this great Earth Mother communicates through metaphor, leveraging the cycles and creatures of the natural world as symbolic teachers and offerings.

In addition to the relationship to the Earth Mother, a strong sense of community plays a pivotal role within the Mexican culture and the indigenous world. Rather than celebrating autonomy or fierce independence, these people derive strength from the support of the village in which they live. That core experience of community is punctuated by ritual celebrations, practices, and ceremonies. These acts—small, daily rituals as well as grand celebrations and deep ceremonial experiences—thread reverence into daily life. And among all the things that are celebrated and viewed as sacred, perhaps the most revered of all is childhood. The wild spirits innate to children are fostered and encouraged in these cultures, rather than suppressed or controlled.

The indigenous use of psychedelic medicines is relevant and essential to our discussion here, because the indigenous communities that work with plant medicines are most intimately familiar with how they communicate and function. We *must* talk sensitively about this indigenous wisdom and their methods within a clinical context, because we must learn from their ancient wisdom and not appropriate it.

In this book, I braid together what I've learned over the last five years of observing indigenous and Mexican curanderas and practitioners, and the foundational and ongoing training I've gleaned from eight years of studying within the clinical framework(s) of psychedelic-assisted therapy. This marriage of science and spirit is critical to the future potential of psychedelic healing. When we bring together the wisdom of these two worlds where science and metaphysics meet, we can truly heal.

Science and Spirit

Historically, science and spirit have been in opposition. One seeks to quantify and explain, while the other seeks to transcend. But no one wins when only one person or perspective can be right. We must combine the best of these approaches in a way that is tailored to each individual to have the greatest impact.

When the recent pandemic hit, the world and my inbox blew up. I was not advertising that I was working as a guide, but I knew that I wanted to move in that direction. I was also deeply humbled by the gravity of the work and grappling with my own imposter syndrome. While I was well-educated and now see the relevance of everything I studied as preparation for my role as a psychedelic therapist, parts of me felt inadequate because I lacked a conventional clinical background. I had more than ten years of professional experience as an executive-level coach working in human and professional development at big organizations. No doubt I could support people. I'd been doing it for years, arguably all my life, starting first with my parents. But the gravitas of this work in the psychedelic world felt much more sacred, more vulnerable, more tenuous.

Although many success stories were making headlines, there were also horror stories of things gone wrong—stories of re-traumatization, of violation, of people getting seriously hurt all in the name and space of healing. Given everything in the not-so-distant cultural history of psychedelics, I became quickly and deliberately focused on the topic of harm-reduction. How do we bring this body of work forward in the safest and most effective ways? How do we honor that most baseline fundamental law of care: *Do no harm.*

One answer to this dilemma lay in significantly more clinical training. While planting roots and nurturing a garden of growth in our new Mexican home, I completed two essential trainings within a therapeutic model called Internal Family Systems (IFS) developed by Richard Schwartz. The IFS model is based on the premise that inside each of us is an internal family that is built up through traumatic experiences to ensure protection from harm to the most vulnerable parts inside us. It also deals with "legacy burdens," something akin to intergenerational trauma. Both these concepts were instrumental in my understanding of how to work with integrity and skill within the psychedelic space.

Moreover, the more I studied, the more I understood the subtle, but significant, distinction between being "trauma-aware" and "trauma-trained." This understanding led me to an intensive course on the treatment of trauma facilitated by some of the most respected voices in the field—Bessel van der Kolk, Pat Ogden, Janina Fisher, Stephen Porges, and Peter Levine, to name a few. My motivation for this rapid consumption of content circles back to harm-reduction. As articles and podcasts presented more accounts of people being harmed in the psychedelic space, it became clear that having an awareness of how trauma impacts the psyche may be a great starting point, but it is not nearly enough.

Around this time, I discovered the renowned podcast "Back from the Abyss," hosted by Dr. Craig Heacock. Heacock was a participating therapist in the Phase 3 clinical trials for PTSD treatment with MDMA. He brings a wealth of knowledge acquired over decades to the psychedelic-assisted therapy conversation. I eagerly awaited the release of each new episode and listened immediately. I analyzed, took notes, and then began to reach out to him with questions.

Days before Christmas, I was driving down a bumpy road in Mexico listening to an episode of this podcast in which a woman described a volatile, unsafe relationship she had with her biological father—something I related to deeply. Heacock's therapeutic offering for her was something along the lines of a "parentectomy"—a kind of intense moment in which the child inside this grown woman, stunted by her father's abuse, could be seen and validated, and then step forward into the present.

Moved to tears, I pulled off the road to listen to the rest of the story. Three things became clear in that moment. First, this work of *transference* was at the core of what makes psychedelic-assisted therapy most effective, and it was not understood nearly enough. And I realized that this was an experience I needed more of inside myself to be able to hold that space for others. In fact, transference explained much of what was already happening in my growing practice.

After this experience, I made a vulnerable, but necessary, decision to spend a week of immersive transferential work with Heacock in person. Given the nature of my own father wound, this week felt like decades of talk therapy. In the mornings, as I walked from my rented room to his clinic, I felt like a girl on her way to meet with a transferentially assigned paternal figure. Sometimes I felt as if I were five years old, sometimes like fifteen; sometimes I was scared, sometimes I was giddy. I had never even considered the need to grieve the profound loss of having no emotional connection to one of my parents. In literal terms, of course, Dr. Heacock was not my father, but that was not the point or the goal. The point was that the neurogenesis facilitated by the psychedelic medicines and their unique capacity to dissolve innate fear responses combined with this transferential dynamic to create an opening in which my nervous system and self-concept began to reconsolidate.

For years, I'd heard people talk about the "somatic body." I knew this meant physical, felt experience. But as someone who battled my body and felt largely locked in my brain, this concept remained abstract for me. This work with psychedelics, expanded through transference, catalyzed an increased capacity to feel my body as opposed to simply living in my analytical mind. All the experts say some version of the same thing, but Bessel van der Kolk perhaps said it best: "The body remembers what the mind works hard to forget."[5] It was only with the aid of psychedelics and transference that my body and mind at last began stitching together.

The experience of the week with Dr. Heacock was far more somatically defined than intellectually understood. As the most vulnerable child parts within me were held within a safe, transferential dynamic, I was able to have a corrective experience in which my physical body started to release traumatic memories and feelings stored within—almost without effort. While my logical mind searched for language and insights to explain the experience, my primal body took the lead. In the evenings in my room, I experienced flu-like symptoms. My physical body alternated between shivering with chills and sweating. I had no fever and wasn't physically ill, but I was experiencing a kind of healing reaction somatically through my body. I cried. I laughed. I cried some more. And most important, for the first time in my life, I let my body do its thing.

When this mind-body connection was made clear to me, I knew I wanted to work more intentionally at the somatic level. This led me to become certified as a psychedelic somatic therapist. An integral part of the training involved in this certification is experiential. It is hard, if not impossible, to guide someone through an experience you have not felt yourself. In the experiential part of the training, I came to understand how the autonomic nervous system works and how to leverage emotions activated in the transferential space to generate somatic release. That physiological release felt something like losing twenty pounds and/or gaining tons of new bandwidth in my brain.

These are the primary modalities, trainings, and processes I draw from in my practice with clients. They are informed by deliberate, intensive study and a personal exploration of the experience. The process is anything but glamorous and is far less immediately magical than what the emerging pop culture might suggest. But the healing that is made possible through this therapy is truly incredible, especially when navigated with continuity of care, intention, and holistic support.

The Bones of This Book

This book uses personal experience and real-life accounts to open readers up to the opportunities for integration made possible through psychedelic-assisted therapy. It is intended to help readers discover the great promise that these drugs are showing in current practice. It discusses a variety of medicinal tools and explains how and why they are used. Woven into these discussions are practices and wisdom from indigenous and Mexican healers. Each chapter ends with writing prompts and journaling exercises that are intended to be useful for those working with therapists, as well as for those who are not.

The book consists of three parts that reflect the clinical arc of a psychedelic healing journey: Preparation, Ceremony, and Integration. The first recounts how my own experiences led me to the possibilities of psychedelic-assisted healing. The second uses the stories of real-life patients to illustrate the practice of psychedelic-assisted therapy. The third highlights the enormous healing potential of this journey.

Throughout the book, you will find recurring themes that are tailored to the respective stage of the healing process. For instance, in part I, we'll explore the difference between intentions and unconscious expectations. In part II, you'll learn how ceremony is anchored in intentions that act as a compass to steady your course. In Part III, you'll discover how unconscious expectations can shape and drive the healing process.

My goal is to take you through each stage of the healing arc and give you tools that can help you deepen your own journey through healing. The stories reveal a wide variety of traumatic wounds, but the primary focus is on working with PTSD and CPTSD in conjunction with psychedelic-assisted therapy as a means for full recovery and transformation. I also address which medicinal tools were applied and why. Since my training and experience include working with MDMA, psilocybin, ketamine, and cannabis, these are the tools you'll find in the stories.

As I write, ketamine is already legal across the United States, while cannabis and psilocybin are rapidly following. MDMA is projected to be on the legal list within the next year. At this writing, there is a delay in the FDA approval process. This is another socio-political response that mirrors the last war on drugs. The consensus is that things are still moving forward with approval, but delayed. As we make rapid, accelerated strides toward the complete legalization of this work in clinical settings, more and more people are reaching out in urgent need of help. But while legalization is exciting, it also poses great challenges and inevitably will inflate costs, making these therapies impossible for many to afford. My hope is that the stories in this book, while not the same as having a personal guide, can provide readers with information, tools, and support to educate them and empower them as they consider this journey. As Brené Brown said: "Stories are data with a soul."[6] As much as we want to quantify the science and know the results, we are starved for real-life examples.

I tell my clients that one person somewhere along the way who is securely attached can save a life. It could be a grandparent, a teacher, a cousin, a friend. It really doesn't matter who. It only matters that they were there, that they listened, that they showed up, that they provided some sense of safety and the hope that unconditional love is real. While a book can never be a substitute for a skilled therapist holding such an important space, if the contents of these pages provide comfort and safety in your journey from pain to transformation, then my heart is grateful and the stories have served their purpose.

I'll be working with the medicines for as long as I'm on this planet—working with love and intention to help others safely navigate this healing journey. If that work can help you remember who you are, help you believe you are enough, help you learn to love and laugh at yourself inside the magical mess, that's my reward. I'll be right here with you throughout your journey. And remember that the worst is already behind you and the path forward can be free and clear.

PART I

Preparation

As long as you keep secrets and suppress information, you are fundamentally at war with yourself. . . . The critical issue is allowing yourself to know what you know. That takes an enormous amount of courage.

— Bessel van der Kolk

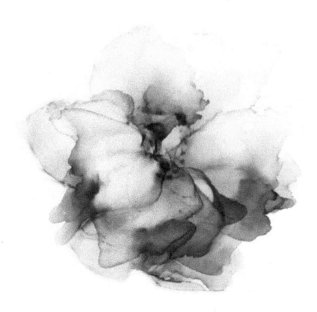

(1)

The Pilgrimage
for Proof

Trauma comes back as a reaction, not a memory.

— Bessel van der Kolk

A PILGRIMAGE IS DEFINED AS A LONG JOURNEY to somewhere sacred made as an act of devotion. Thus there is no more perfect word to describe the psychedelic journey to reclaim ourselves from the abyss of violence, abandonment, and abuse.

On the pilgrimage for proof, deep in the psychedelic realms of the subconscious, we discover the parts of our story that are hidden from ourselves. Most survivors of PTSD and CPTSD share a common struggle. Their memories of childhood are foggy at best, if not entirely inaccessible. This can be a major impediment to healing in conventional therapy. What is there to talk about if the memories can't be found?

Survivors struggling to feel safe, who have been disempowered by abuse, default to believing the dominant narrative of the family system in which they were raised. But the version of history told by the abuser is full of secrets, shame, gaslighting, and lies, and it's easy to get lost inside the dissonance of the stories we're told and lose touch with the truth of what our bodies know. The persistent conditioning of abuse makes it all but impossible to trust.

Having navigated the pilgrimage for proof myself and with numerous clients, I have come to understand the notion of repressed memories in an entirely different way. As memories emerge in the medicine space, they come with the realization that they were never fully absent. Like a phantom limb that aches even though it's gone, our memories linger in the mind, but are anesthetized from feeling. In the psychedelic space, we experience the medicine's capacity to stitch those memories and our bodies back together. A memory of the body touched inappropriately; an abortion following an incident of rape; the sudden, traumatic loss of secure attachment to a child, a parent, or a caregiver; the violent divorce of parents—all these memories and the images connected to them come back to be the center of our focus from an archive buried deep in the mind. As the memories return, so does a deeply felt somatic sense in the body.

This felt sense is an altogether different kind of knowing that is reflected, not through thought, but rather through embodied experience. Gradually, each individual's search for concrete, empirical details gives way to an awakening of what has been buried. This might surface as discoveries like:

» "Oh my god. I didn't realize how terrified I was. I feel that now."

» "I still don't regret my decision, but there's all this pain I had no idea existed."

» "I can feel my devastation. The grief is crushing. How did I never notice this before?"

» "I can see now how alone I was—how I had to basically become a grown-up overnight."

In the earliest stages of our pilgrimage for proof, it is difficult to trust these returning memories. What is clear in the medicine space is sometimes difficult to hold on to in everyday life. We struggle to maintain that new-felt sense of knowing and connection to ourselves. The historical stories start to return, their familiarity bringing a kind of dark comfort despite the dissonance that surrounds them. The minute we challenge history, everything requires reevaluation. That is a daunting prospect.

Psychedelic-assisted therapy requires time, patience, and support. The emerging cultural mythology that psychedelics are the newest quick cure for trauma invites even greater potential for disappointment and despair. Our culture of immediacy has lost touch with what it means to surrender, to wait in patience and trust. Psychedelic healing has the potential to reconnect us to a more abundant and less instantaneous pace of life. But we must be willing to do the work and wait for the results to unfold.

If we hold a steady course on this pilgrimage, the promise of trust gradually returns. Fear and doubt give way to new growth and possibility. We stop perpetually seeking proof outside of ourselves and look for truth within our bodies. And we begin to honor the sacred within ourselves.

YOUR TURN

What therapies or treatments have you tried before considering psychedelics? Of the things you tried that were helpful, what commonalities do they share? Were they somatic? Cathartic? Creative? Look for a pattern of things that have resonated with your body and your brain.

A Village of Care

I've yet to meet a person embarking on the path of psychedelic therapy who hasn't already tried many other modalities. Rather, I hear a common refrain that sounds something like this: "I've tried everything. I'm desperate to feel better." This is the essence of what draws people to this path—some combination of desperation, hope, and a sense of purpose.

An integral part of preparing for the pilgrimage for proof and the psychedelic journey is understanding that it will change *everything*. How we see our families, our culture, and even ourselves—all of this will look different on the other side of the journey. Preparing for this deconstruction requires strange internal acrobatics in which we orient ourselves to an ephemeral experience that resists definition. Naturally, clients ask: "How do I prepare myself for the unknown?"

Truthfully, we can't be entirely prepared. We can't know until we begin what is buried in our subconscious. But we can step into the process with conscious consent and intention, understanding that things are likely to feel harder before they get easier. We can prepare ourselves to start over, as forbidding as that may sound.

In healthy anticipation of beginning again, we cultivate better tools and allow ourselves to be held within what I call a *village of care*. We've all heard the adage that it takes a village to raise a child. It takes an even mightier village to resuscitate wounded children who are haunted by neglect and abuse. I'll talk more about the village of care throughout the book. For now, suffice it to say that we must understand that, to break deeply entrenched cycles of abuse and limiting beliefs, it is essential to provide in the present the support we longed for as children.

As we prepare ourselves for this pilgrimage by cultivating tools and conscious community, we start to understand how loyalty to those who hurt us created a rupture inside. Repairing that rupture requires that we reclaim our stories. In so doing, we may lose friends and family members. We may find that speaking our truth is seen as an act of betrayal. But we must be willing to upset others to save ourselves. A village of care buoys us in the face of that reality.

Think of yourself as being like any voyager on a quest. To prepare yourself for the unknown, you gather resources and build strength to move beyond any obstacles you may encounter. You prepare for challenges proactively—not to will them into being, but so that your resolve is not shaken when they occur. When you are scapegoated by family, or told you're too sensitive, or even called a liar, you can surrender into the care of the village you've cultivated and hold fast to the resources around you to forge new pathways. In so doing, you cut the cords of the past and find your way out of the rupture and into the present. Even with all this intention and awareness, however, we're not insulated from pain. We are just equipped to face it and feel it in corrective ways.

This book will take you on a journey that mirrors the arc of the psychedelic path from preparation, to ceremony, to integration. Every chapter reflects a microcosm of that arc, so that wherever you land in its pages, you can walk away with a felt sense of what is possible and what is involved. My goal is to immerse you in all the core elements of this journey and help deepen your understanding of the metaphorical language the medicine speaks. I will be your invested, empathic guide, offering direction, relevant exercises, and support. In the experiences of others who've traversed the pilgrimage for proof and made it to the other side, you will see how cycles can be broken. You will learn it is possible, even if daunting, to build a blueprint for a different life—a life in which science and spirit meet and the impossible becomes possible.

JOURNAL PROMPTS AND REFLECTIONS

» Consider the notion of a pilgrimage for proof in terms of felt senses in the body rather than concrete details. Write about what your senses feel or don't feel.

» Many survivors suspect they have repressed memories. This is often because they're not as far away as they tell themselves. Consider some of the most recurring images from your childhood. Bring curiosity to those memories, either in meditation or journaling, and reflect on what comes up.

» What do you feel you most need to prove? To whom? And why?

» How do you feel about your responses to these questions now that you've heard/seen yourself express them out loud or written them on paper?

2

Epigenetics and Intergenerational Trauma

Sleeping inside each of our ancestors
were fragments of traumas too great
to be resolved in one generation.

— Mark Wolynn

MY DAD CRIED WHEN I WAS BORN because I wasn't a boy. I heard this story over and over as I was growing up. My father disliked girls and women because he had been rejected by his own mother and taught by his father that women fell into one of two categories—whores, who were tools of utility and occasional pleasure, and wives, who were servants to a patriarchal order established to ensure a man's legacy.

My father came from scarcity, repression, and rage. He lived a life that was permeated by moonshine, sadness, and sex. Sex without love. Sex as sin. Sex as a release of shame and rage. He knew nothing of a life of unencumbered love and connection.

My budding breasts and curves emerged early and with force, catching everyone by surprise. I started taping them down when I turned ten in a desperate attempt to keep them secret. I was hyper-aware of the attention they drew and the negative impressions that attention might give about me. I did everything I could think of to make myself smaller than I was. I was groomed for objectification in a church where both the gift and art of my body were seen as sin, abominations to be handled firmly, with conviction. This meant that my body and my sexuality were problems to solve, not worlds to explore.

I observed friends with their fathers, seeing how they looked at their daughters with affection. This was foreign to me. My dad's experience of me was marked by anxiety and disdain. Ensuring my purity was simply another burden to carry. Our dynamic was bound up in this movement between love and hate, vulnerability and shame, right and wrong. We languished in a tug of war between annihilation and possibility.

Most of my twenties and thirties were spent trying to resuscitate my colonized body back to life. I took medication and went to therapy. I got better, but many things remained broken inside. I folded these broken aspects of myself like winter clothes that you put away when summer comes and tucked them so far back in the closet of my mind that I almost forgot they were there—until I gave birth to my son.

After he was born, the emaciated, eighteen-year-old, stack-of-bones version of myself who was incapable of self-love re-emerged, begging to be parented and seen. She smelled of honeysuckle and, when she wasn't crying, she hummed "Amazing Grace" through a trembling jaw. I tried everything to quiet her noise. My therapist suggested eye-movement desensitization and reprocessing therapy, (EMDR), but the girl with rattling bones scoffed. Tired of being repressed, she demanded that I listen. I knew that, if I was going to raise a son who would grow up to be a man who honored women, I had to first love and forgive myself. But I had no idea yet how to do that.

Meet Vigilance

Desperate for rest and peace, I found a therapist in a robust network of underground practitioners who specialized in these kinds of wounds. Six weeks later, weaned from anti-anxiety and depression meds, I arrived at her studio in the woods. I sipped a mug of teal-green psilocybin tea. It smelled like earth and tasted like dirt. And this is where I met a part of me I call *Vigilance*.

As the medicine began to work its way through my cells, I felt a sharp, tingling sensation, like when your foot falls asleep and then wakes. I felt this tingling from the crown of my head to the tips of my toes and everywhere in between—as if something dead were resurrecting in my womb space. Then Vigilance appeared as an awakening from numbness. She was five. She was seven. She was running and hiding, terrified of everything—especially of being dirty. She scrubbed her hands and her body, hoping to wash away a filth and shame that had been passed down the generational line.

I saw my father as well. But not as my father. I saw him as a five-year-old little boy, running, chased through the fields of his boyhood. He was another version of Vigilance. The blueprint inside was both different and the same. That's when I realized that we were both casualties of a war neither of us wanted to fight. I faced this man-boy across a great expansive field as a girl turned mother—standing with my son on my hip. My father stared back. We stood like stair steps of possibility, like a continuum of hurt to hope. The promise of innocence. The tragedy of childhood lost to unresolved pain.

Inside Vigilance, underneath her rattling bones, lived my voice, my orgasm, my creativity, my rage, and the deepest essence of my love. My power pulsed from her pain. And the path forward became clear. The pain story had to end with me. Together with my son, we left those blighted fields and stepped into the golden sun, never looking back.

Vigilance used to be a bird with clipped wings living in a cage. But not anymore.

YOUR TURN

Consider your family of origin. What do you know and understand already about your history and your trauma? What are you (consciously or unconsciously) working to forget?

Ancestral Pain

The narrative at the start of this chapter reflects an awareness that emerged as I started my own psychedelic healing journey. This journey awakened my understanding of the entrenched layers of epigenetic and intergenerational trauma in my family system. The beliefs that haunted me were inherited, not unlike my skin tone or my eye color. Beginning to see the origin of my pain as outside of myself and not entirely my fault was a catalyst for change. That understanding became the seedling of self-empathy from which my deepest transformation grew.

In my work now with clients, this is a critical part of our larger preparation conversation. With curiosity and transparency, we investigate the generational archives of what each parent and grandparent brought to the equation. People are often surprised—and, in some ways, relieved—to see that the pattern didn't begin with them and that the burden of responsibility doesn't all rest on their shoulders.

Research has revealed that our life experiences have the capacity to affect the expression of our genes. This means that the old belief that our genetics are pre-determined and immutable no longer holds true. It means that the topic of "nature vs. nurture"—the consideration of the impact of trauma and how it travels through generations—demands even more psychological, developmental study. Historically, we've seen our genes as the hardware that determines who we are. Epigentics, on the other hand, is understood to be the software that operates at a level above the DNA itself. But as we update and upgrade our "epigenetic software," science and data have shown that the hardware itself—our genetic make-up—also begins to change.

When clients bring an awareness and understanding of the impact of epigenetics into the depths of the psychedelic journey, it helps validate what might otherwise feel like blind hope. Knowing that things need to change is the essential first step. Understanding that those needed changes are likely rooted far back in history can alleviate the sting of feeling singularly responsible and irreparably broken. Rather, we can tap into the possibility that our healing has the potential to alter the composition of our lineage.

JOURNAL PROMPTS AND REFLECTIONS

» What keeps you awake at night? What would it feel like if those things weren't there?

» What limiting beliefs, manic/OCD tendencies, or disordered thinking are getting in the way of your fulfillment? How are you managing these things now?

» How would you like this to be different than it is? How would you like it to feel differently than it does?

» Who in your family or childhood displays similar tendencies?

3

Index Events

*I am not what happened to me, I am
what I choose to become. . . . Until you
make the unconscious conscious, it will
direct your life and you will call it fate.*

— Carl Jung

AS A THERAPIST, when I begin a psychedelic healing journey with
clients, one of the first activities I have them complete is a timeline of
events. I ask them to mark anything of significance on this timeline—good
or bad, or possibly even something that doesn't make logical sense, like
a recurring intrusive thought or a nightmare. As we look through this
timeline, we begin to see the defining moments that are often referred to
as "index events"—the moment(s) or point(s) at which their sense of self
began to splinter due to trauma.

An index event that had a significant impact on me was a severe car accident I had when I was sixteen—one that could have taken my life but somehow,
miraculously, did not. It happened at the peak of my struggle with anorexia.
Over the course of that summer, I'd gone from 125 to eighty-seven pounds.
My hair was falling out in chunks. My menstrual cycle had stopped. I was surviving on 500 to 600 calories a day and had successfully made it to a size zero.

The day of the accident, I wove in and out of consciousness due to malnourishment. Floating stars were the last thing I saw before waking up to the car spiraling across the road. I'd hit a patch of water from a thunderstorm and the car hydroplaned. The fleeting thought that I might die flashed through my mind. I wondered how badly the impact would hurt and if perhaps death was the best way to escape. These thoughts shattered as the car crashed into a barbed-wire fence with intense force and toppled upside down into the middle of a cow pasture.

As the wild motion came to a screeching halt, everything became painfully still. The image of my grandfather, who'd passed of cancer just three months before, appeared before me. His love saved my life. His death woke me up from a trauma-induced trance. When his face first came into form after the crash, I thought for a minute that I had already died. I thought he was waiting to receive me, the same way he had waited for me by the door of his house when I was little girl.

But then I heard his voice. "You get up and out of this car. You get out of this broken place, and you make something of your life. *This is not all there is*," he said firmly, intently. Then his face faded away.

Smoke billowed out from under the hood of the car. Instinct, adrenaline, and my grandfather's words coursed through my body. I used my backpack to knock out the window and slithered out between shards of glass. I crawled up the ravine onto the street, where a string of firetrucks and an ambulance had already arrived. An elderly couple who lived nearby had seen the whole thing and called 911. They came over to me, wrapped a blanket around my shoulders, and invited me to come inside. Disoriented and shaky, I walked with them toward their house, glancing over my shoulder once to see a burst of flames light up the sky.

"You made it out just in time, honey," the man said with a kind of nurturing concern that felt largely foreign to me. "Now let's go call your parents and get you home."

"We can't call my parents," I replied adamantly. "They'll be furious."

After assuring me that my parents would be happy I was okay, they gave me a soft drink. I can still recall its fizz and how I didn't care about the calories it contained. I remember thinking that maybe I could just stay there indefinitely—there, in the kindness of strangers.

I don't remember anything after that, certainly not talking to the police. I can't tell you what I said to them because it's all blurry. I can't say if one or both of my parents came to get me. I don't recall the car ride home or what anyone said about the accident. I was haunted by the swirl of motion and the utter loss of control.

Prior to the car wreck, I'd spent every ounce of my energy trying to be perfect. Perfection was required to keep my dad's rage at bay, and to give my mother a sense of happiness. I'm sure this was not their intent, but it was the message I internalized all the same. If I could be perfect, then there could be peace. Without perfection, home felt like an emotional war zone. When perfection and starving myself failed, an overarching sense of desperation led me to explore things I never would have considered before.

First Steps

My first introduction to psychedelics came shortly after that crash—admittedly not in a therapeutic space. Psychedelic therapy was nowhere on anyone's radar in the Bible Belt in the early 1990s. Having been raised as an evangelical Christian, I had been conditioned to fear everything—even myself. Despite that, I had plenty of hippie musician friends in Nashville, Tennessee, who smoked pot and ate mushrooms.

What surprised me most was how those forbidden things—like marijuana, mushrooms, and MDMA—awakened a sense of hope and love I'd never felt. While I lacked the guidance and support of a therapist to help me navigate my psychedelic experiences, as part of my eating-disorder recovery, I was required to meet weekly with a psychiatrist and a nutritionist.

The psychiatrist in charge of my case had a short, boyish haircut and dressed in a masculine-style suit. We were required to attend the first appointment with her as a family. The over-arching message was that an eating disorder happens to the family, not just the individual suffering. My dad screamed the whole way there about how everyone was going to blame him and how ungrateful we all were. He lasted fifteen minutes before bursting out the door of the psychiatrist's office in a fit of rage. Mom crumpled in tears. I stared at the doctor, waiting to see how she would handle this. I don't remember what she said, but I remember more screaming and crying in the car on the way home. I remember thinking that even the "helpers" couldn't help. I longed for a way to escape.

That was the last session my dad attended. "I'm not going to listen to any goddamn woman dressed like a man tell me about my problems," he ranted. After a few more visits with my mother, the doctor suggested that I come alone. I was required to gain weight and meet with her weekly, and was threatened with being sent to an in-patient care facility if I didn't. During those meetings, it occurred to me that this eating disorder/best friend had turned on me. My body had forgotten how to digest food. I had to learn to eat all over again, like a baby.

The most confusing part of all this was how, during the whole summer leading up to this crisis, my father had praised me for my discipline. "You never want to be fat like your mom," he said. To be anything other than skinny was to give someone permission to abuse you. To be fat was to be utterly unlovable.

About six months into my treatment, the doctor gave me a list of behaviors, words, and actions that were unacceptable for my father. Her list included things like name-calling, threatening to hurt me, screaming violently, or threatening my mother. She looked at me through thick-rimmed glasses and said: "If he breaks any one of these rules, you call my cell at any hour of the day. I will make it stop." I walked out of that office with a feeling I'd never had before. Now, I had the promise of protection—an actual boundary.

I knew it was only a matter of time, and, sure enough, a couple of days later I came home three minutes past curfew. My dad was waiting, screaming, blood boiling, veins popping out of his forehead—familiar father rage. But this time, I walked to the phone. My mom cried and screamed in the background, pleading for me to stop. I dialed the afterhours number, heart racing. He stood glaring, in shock that I had the audacity to challenge his authority. The doctor's voice came on the other end of the line: "Micah, are you ok?" she asked in her stern voice.

"He's threatening to hurt me," I said.

"Put your father on the phone. I need to speak with him right now. I'll see you Friday in my office," she said, matter of factly, just like that—as if it were no big deal. I'd been waiting seventeen years for someone to make him stop threatening me. I handed him the phone and stood close enough to hear.

"Mr. Stover, you're going to need to step back and calm down. If you cannot control your temper and are abusive with your words or hands, I will call the police. Can I count on you not to make this worse?" she asked. Trembling, I stared at him. He had loathing in his eyes, astounded that I had the nerve to protect myself and defy him.

"There's no need for any police around here," he grumbled and hung up the phone before skulking to his room.

That was the last time he verbally threatened my safety. I moved out of their house shortly after, enrolled in a university, and then moved to Asia to study and teach. But there was something about that combination—a car crash, a near-death brush with fate, extensive therapy, a sprinkling of psychedelics, and someone strong enough to set a boundary—that gave me exactly what I needed to have the courage to leave it all behind. In university, I committed all the energy I'd given to my eating disorder to academics. I decided that being smart was better than being pretty. I left and didn't go back for five years.

YOUR TURN

What is your earliest memory of feeling unsafe in your body? Many children in abusive homes think their experience is "normal" and develop a host of adaptive/maladaptive ways to cope with their stress. In what ways do you recall managing your emotions as a child? As an adolescent? Now? What is your relationship to those coping mechanisms? Do you still rely on them when anxiety, stress, or depression emerge?

In psychedelic-assisted therapy, the ailment or issue that brings people to the process is rarely the beginning of their struggles. Usually, in cases of PTSD and CPTSD, the trauma is buried and camouflaged deep in the person's memory and nervous system. I hadn't considered that car wreck for years, until I started my psychedelic journey. But it is clear in hindsight how everything about my life hinged on that incident.

JOURNAL PROMPTS AND REFLECTIONS

» Consider your personal timeline. What are the moments, memories, and events that stand out—good or bad. Are they logical or seemingly random? At what ages did they occur?

» Collect pictures of yourself at those respective ages. What do you see in those pictures?

» Write a story about one of those memories as if you were telling it about a character other than yourself. How does the narrative change when you remove yourself from the story?

4

Set and Setting

*When working with psychedelics, we
must consider the state of mind as
well as the environment in order to
have a transformative experience.*

— Timothy Leary

THE TERMS "SET" AND "SETTING" GET TOSSED AROUND a lot in
the therapy world—often casually and without clarity. "Set" refers to the
mindset in which you enter the psychedelic experience. "Setting" refers to
the container, the environment, in which that happens. There isn't a one-
size-fits-all, right or wrong set or setting. Rather, it is important that conscious consideration be given to whatever configuration makes the most
sense for each individual based on the nature of their trauma. This became
abundantly clear to me in my interaction with Callie.

Callie's Struggle

The first time I met Callie was in an integration circle. I had recently fin-
ished an apprenticeship and over a year of self-study with the medicines.
My family and I were newly relocated to Mexico, and, while I knew there

was an indigenous world of medicine work now at my fingertips, I had no idea how to tap into that community.

During the integration circle, in which a small group from the underground psychedelic community met online, Callie was visibly distraught. As people shared their experiences, she struggled to hold eye contact. Her body was visibly trembling. She moved from inside her house to outside— back and forth—trying frantically to find a spot to settle. She switched her video on and off. When I saw her face, she was clearly crying.

What struck me most was that the facilitator said absolutely nothing. The participants in the group said nothing. There was zero acknowledgment of a giant elephant in the room. We were gathered to talk about trauma and abandonment wounds. Meanwhile, one of the participants was visibly struggling and no one said anything.

As the hour passed, I felt increasingly sad and concerned for Callie and baffled by the larger group dynamic. The whole purpose was support, but I didn't see a lot of support being given. I found myself in a community, but was struck by how isolated and disconnected it felt. This raised a lot of questions for me about the efficacy of group work in general when it comes to trauma, at least in the earliest stages of the healing process.

We had all shared contact details at the start of the virtual circle. I hesitated, having never met Callie outside of this interaction, but somehow I couldn't stop thinking about her. Her words that reverberated most strongly for me were: "I don't feel safe. I'm so alone. I'm scared for myself."

From a trauma standpoint, this is something you can't take lightly. And I also knew that it can be legitimately hard to manage the range of human experiences within a group context. I wondered if the facilitator followed up with her. I wondered if anyone was going to be in touch with her. Did she have a therapist, a family member, or a friend, anyone who would be checking in? After a few hours of debating, I sent her a message.

"Hi Callie. I was in the integration circle today. I've been thinking about you. I hope you have support. I know healing is hard and lonely. If you need someone to talk to you, you can call me."

My phone lit up with a reply even before I put it down on the counter.

"Oh my god, thank you for reaching out! I'm having a really hard time. It would help a lot to talk to someone if you're willing. Let me know a good time."

We spoke the next morning.

Many Paths—Different Needs

As Callie shared her story with me, I learned she'd had a painful experience in the medicine space. She'd found her therapist through the underground community and local meet-up groups for psychedelic support. The therapist she'd worked with had a great reputation in the community, lots of relevant credentials, and over two decades of clinical practice. Professionally speaking, she seemed solid.

Despite that, Callie's experience with her in the medicine space was one that unintentionally reinforced core abandonment wounds and attachment injuries. The facilitator had given Callie a heroic dose in her first session that had taken her to a pre-verbal, early-infancy state of abandonment. She couldn't access language during her session to articulate how terrified she felt—not then or even three months later.

Although the facilitator was more or less present for the majority of the session, she made minimal attempts to engage Callie. When she tried at one point to say she was struggling, the facilitator firmly instructed her to put on eye shades and trust the process. She told her to stop resisting the experience, but beyond this directive, didn't engage.

At one point, Callie, who was curled up in a fetal position, recalled peeking out from the eye shades to see if the facilitator was still there. The child inside was terrified of abandonment. While the therapist had not intended that Callie experience a re-traumatization of this kind, that is exactly what happened. Callie told me she remained writhing in the fetal position for several more hours before being put in a taxi and sent home. There was no resolution. She was still in this dysregulated state two weeks later, when she attended the integration call where we'd met.

Over the following months, I learned that Callie's biological mother had struggled with mental-health issues and had been emotionally unavailable most of her life before passing at a young age due to addiction. Callie had come to psychedelic-assisted therapy to heal this maternal abandonment wound, which was then inadvertently reinforced. While not precisely the facilitator's intention or fault, this dynamic happens far too often without a corrective experience.

These are the scenarios we *must* talk about, because they illuminate the intersection where everything that could have gone right ended up going wrong instead. What is most concerning is how accidentally this can happen. Just as our parents did the "best they could," it takes more than positive intent and a good heart to avoid making a mess. When we step into the psychedelic-assisted therapy space to support people with complex trauma, it is imperative that we are informed of the trauma we are addressing and truly understand the complexity of attachment wounds that will emerge in the psychedelic state.

In Callie's case, she intentionally selected to work with a trained therapist with the medicines following a clinical model. She chose this path after extensive research and discussions with lots of friends who'd also embarked on psychedelic healing journeys. For Callie, the clinical model promised a sense of security and structure that felt aligned with her early attachment trauma. Though she respected the indigenous path many friends had taken, she was reticent to take her wounds "into the jungle" with a group of strangers. Given her struggle to engage in the integration circle, it was not surprising that individual work felt less overwhelming.

She explained through tears: "I thought I was doing the right thing. I considered going to Peru or Costa Rica. I know that's the origin of these medicines. It worked for my friends. But my intuition said I needed something different. Somehow, I still got it wrong."

Callie felt she'd made a mistake when, in actuality, she was right on several counts. First, she was right to listen to her intuition, to trust her knowingness that one-on-one support was what she needed. She was also correct that indigenous people have been working with plant medicines longer than we've had established clinical practices. Their approaches and relationship to these medicines are categorically different. This doesn't mean that those of us outside the indigenous community can't benefit from their methods and wisdom. Quite the contrary. But to expect to arrive in their world and be transformed by the medicine in a matter of days is unrealistic. For a person coming from an activated state of PTSD, the jarring nature of this transition could be re-traumatizing as opposed to healing.

Given the complexity, you may be asking yourself: How do I know I'm on the right track? How do I know what set and setting are right for me? What if I listen to my intuition, make a conscious choice to follow a particular path—as Callie did—and still find myself in a painful, retraumatizing situation? These are necessary questions that anyone considering psychedelic-assisted therapy must explore.

Finding Alignment

Selecting the right set and setting comes down to the profound importance of conscious choice and an intentional and thorough preparation process. The preparation process creates space for holistic health assessment and attunement of each individual's intuition. We must deconstruct the binary thinking that assumes there is a "right" way vs. a "wrong" way to approach this healing path. As we deconstruct this binary model, we can lean into the actuality that everyone needs something a little bit different.

Even with that acknowledgment, we can establish parameters for safety, baselines for conduct, and guardrails for protection. We can agree that this is essential and still surrender rigidity and reductionistic controls that strip individuals of agency and voice. For a culture that defines success in healthcare as controlling symptoms, this is the biggest challenge *and* the greatest opportunity. Psychedelic healing is not a quick fix. It's a commitment to a long journey home to ourselves.

After Callie and I connected a couple times, she asked if I would be open to working with her in the medicine space. Despite a difficult first ceremony, she longed for something corrective and felt an intuitive call to try again. The process so far, even if uncomfortable, had provided some tough lessons about what did and didn't work for her. Her courage and commitment were inspiring. It felt clear that, with more comprehensive preparation and trauma-informed attention to her attachment wounds, the outcome could be different.

Together, we created a plan for her preparation process. We worked for months before incorporating medicines, intentionally building a dynamic of trust and safety. We talked extensively about support in the medicine space if she began to feel overwhelmed or anxious. We created a plan for what medicines, what doses, and what anchors would maintain safety if she became activated.

Integral to the effectiveness of this plan was Callie's sense of agency. For example, could she feel safe to tell me she didn't want to wear eye shades if I made that recommendation? What would she need to feel safe enough to disagree with me, the person holding a transferential place and space of authority? There was no rush to answer these questions and jump to the medicine to fix the pain. Rather, we worked in a measured way to lay a solid foundation. The relational foundation was the key ingredient that helped the medicine work.

--------- **YOUR TURN** ---------

What draws you to this path of healing? What do you already know about psychedelics? What questions or fears do you have? How easy (or hard) is it to access your intuition?

Making Choices

Every day, I am asked how to find the right guide and what medicine and setting to choose. This is one of the most important and difficult questions to examine. It's difficult because, as described above, there is no single right path or answer. It's also hard to discern intuition from fear when people are activated in their trauma. Trauma disconnects us from our intuition, because the very people who should have been safest caused us harm. From that point forward, trusting becomes a challenge.

Despite all this complexity, however, there are clear steps and discernable questions that can help you carve out a path. Here are a few:

» What is the nature of your trauma?

» How old were you when things went awry?

» What was your connection like with your mother and/or father? Siblings? Grandparents? Caregivers?

» Have you had any prior experience(s) with psychedelics? What were they like?

» Do you generally feel better one-on-one or in groups?

» Do you feel as if you understand your past, your childhood? Or is it hard to remember?

» Do you feel more comfortable around males or females? Or are you neutral?

» Have you had therapy before? If so, what worked and what didn't?

» Do you tend to be more controlling and vigilant, or disassociated and lost in your thoughts?

The other critical piece to finding the right guide is remembering that you are ultimately interviewing someone to hold a vulnerable, transformative space for you.

Many people report that one medicine session feels like years of talk therapy. While this is hopeful, it is also important to do the work to integrate those insights. Some clients come to consultations saying they have a million questions, but then struggle to articulate any of them. This is largely the result of attempting to navigate an experience that, at this point, is rarely discussed and only marginally understood. Whether you're someone on your own healing quest or a practitioner considering working in this field, these are great questions to explore during preparation and when interviewing a potential therapist.

- » What is your training to do this work?

- » Have you had psychedelic experiences yourself or only studied the process in training?

- » How long have you been practicing?

- » What did you do before this and how is that relevant?

- » How do you support yourself and maintain boundaries, while also being available to clients as they navigate this process?

- » What is your philosophy as relates to touch?

- » How many clients have you worked with, and do you have any testimonials you can share?

- » What was the most challenging and/or rewarding case you've seen?

- » What inspires you the most about the potential of this therapy?

- » What are the biggest risks and/or your greatest concerns?

Most practitioners offer consultations to assess if you're a good match. Leverage this opportunity to explore the connection. It's important to see how your nervous system responds to the practitioner's presence.

JOURNAL PROMPTS AND REFLECTIONS

» Journal about who in your world felt safest when you were little.

» Try to imagine or picture yourself as a child. Look at old photos if you have them. See if you can tap into what they evoke inside you.

» Find an artifact or talisman of comfort—a lovie or blanket you slept with at night, or a particular book, or a special place. Describe that person, place, or thing with as much detail as you can possibly recall.

5

The Right Medicine

*Our indigenous herbalists say to pay attention
when plants come to you; they're bringing
you something you need to learn.*

— Robin Wall Kimmerer

ONE OF THE QUESTIONS I RECEIVE MOST OFTEN—after how to choose a therapist and setting, that is—is what medicine to incorporate in the treatment. In the chapters that follow, I discuss four psychedelic medicines that I have studied extensively: psilocybin, MDMA, cannabis, and ketamine. There are certainly other medicines in the psychedelic apothecary, but my focus here will be on these four in order to remain within the scope of my experience and training.

Psilocybin, MDMA, and ketamine are all well researched, and the research demonstrates their efficacy in the treatment of PTSD and CPTSD, as well as other trauma-related issues. My focus on these three is also informed by their immediate or proximate accessibility in clinical settings. Ketamine is already fully legal in therapeutic settings. MDMA is slated to be available with prescription sometime in 2024, but, at this writing, there is a delay in the FDA aproval process.. Psilocybin clinics are currently opening all over the United States and the drug has a long history of medicinal use in indigenous cultures. Cannabis is available and legal in dispensaries all over the United States and, with a medical card, in states where it is not yet legal for recreational use.

To determine which medicine is best in any given case, we must carefully consider several variables. First and foremost of these is the age at which the trauma began, as well as the nature of the abuse. Was it violent and life-threatening? Was it severe abandonment and neglect? Were these threats experienced persistently or were they incidental and then resolved? Different wounds and different coping mechanisms require different medicines to heal, and each of these factors brings us closer to an intentional and effective treatment plan. Perhaps a combination of medicines will be needed over time. Most likely, individuals' needs will evolve as they come more out of crisis and into the present.

It's also helpful to consider the archetypal role or roles clients played in their family of origin. Were they *rescuers*—the ones who tried to save the family from all the pain? Were they *scapegoats,* blamed for all the problems? Do they fall into a perpetual state of experiencing life as *victims,* disconnected from a sense of agency and power? Do they see themselves in some way as having become *perpetrators* of more pain toward others? Each of these archetypes, just like each child with a different ailment, requires a different treatment. Just because a medicine is a "good medicine" does not mean it's the "right medicine." Considering the whole picture is vital to attaining the desired outcomes.

In addition to these questions, we need to have a clear sense of individuals' overall physical health. Are there potential contra-indications? Are there prescription medicines involved that could impact the psychedelic journey? Is it safe to move forward with this kind of intense therapy in light of the answers to any of these questions?

In case it's not already clear, let me be explicit. The decision of which medicine is the right medicine is not a decision to be made on impulse. Rather, it demands extensive inquiry and introspection, as well as an honest, practical assessment of the composition of patients' lives. What is the scope of their competing responsibilities? Where and which version of psychedelic therapy is going to fit best into their lives? While these questions may seem more cerebral than intuitive or inspired, from a clinical standpoint, they have dramatic implications for how the therapeutic process goes.

As we move through preparation and assess all these important questions and variables, we also have an opportunity to build out the therapeutic relational dynamic of trust and safety. Those seeking therapy have the chance, when guided through this intentional and measured process, to cultivate a sense of *secure attachment* with the individual who will be holding space for them. This is fundamentally important, because the medicine itself is not the cure. It is the medicine in tandem with the relational repair that gives each of us a chance to rewire our thinking and reconstruct our inner world.

YOUR TURN

Consider what you already know about your history and your trauma. Based on that understanding, what elements or ingredients would support you in feeling safe to surrender to an experience you can't mentally manage and control?

The Inner Healer

As we go through this journey to prepare for what is ultimately unknown, we are able to begin getting to know a very necessary, fundamental part inside ourselves—our intuition or *inner healer*. This wise self, often buried deep within, receives the information provided by a skilled guide or therapist, and is able to start engaging in the healing journey in a subtle, but significantly different, way. Rather than coming to the psychedelic journey from a desperate place, we can walk into that experience with a growing grasp of our own agency.

The foundation of my own practice is built on a hybrid of clinical and indigenous medicines and approaches to working with them. At this point, I've spent an equal amount of time and energy training with clinical practitioners and with *curanderas*, or medicine women, and indigenous healers. While there are definitive differences in these approaches, there are also striking overlaps and parallels. It's the marriage of these two perspectives and the respective wisdom they offer that has the capacity to rehabilitate a spirit that is otherwise lost to trauma.

Shortly after my family moved to Mexico, I began to study and learn from a local *curandera*, an indigenous medicine woman descended from a line of healers trained to work in the psychedelic space with plant medicines. She told me that mushrooms were spirits—"little teachers," she called them, as did Maria Sabina. "They help us remember who we are," she said. She explained how their mycelial network existed to help us heal by reconnecting us to the Earth, to each other, and to ourselves. Because they are viewed as spirits themselves, she said, it's important to feel *called to the medicine*. "It's a little like receiving a message from the Earth Mother," she said. "Imagine your mom calling you home for dinner. It's something like that," she noted matter-of-factly, as I stretched myself to understand.

The curandera spoke about the potential risks of consuming medicines outside of a *right relationship*. "Bad trips happen when spirits aren't ready or supported in doing the work," she told me. "Doesn't mean never, just not yet. We can't come to the jungle, removed from everything hard at home in our lives, ingest a lot of medicine, and expect to be fixed. We have to learn how to live, not for the ceremony, but for how to bring the ceremony back to our lives." Reflecting on her words, I felt conflict inside myself. Her wisdom, her connection to spirit and the Earth was palpable. Mine was not. Yet here I was in her world, doing what seemed to be far more appropriately her work. She sensed my turmoil before I even had a chance to name it.

"Look at the mycelial network. Does it stay in one place, or does it expand and diversify? The answers to all your questions are right there," this wise woman said. "The spirit of the medicine is bigger than you or me. It must travel beyond these roots. The medicine belongs to the Earth, not me or you," she added, after pausing for a minute. I was quiet, taking it all in. Then she hugged me the way a mom hugs an overwhelmed child and brushed her hand over my cheek. "Trust your intentions," she said, smiling.

"If they are pure, then the work is aligned. The challenge is not the movement out of indigenous, but rather, the integrity of heart and spirit with which the medicine is held. Hold the sacred as sacred and be aware of the colonizer. If you do this, you can build bridges we desperately need."

Each day, when I talk with clients about their paths, I hold the wisdom of the curandera in my heart. I stand steady in my clinical training and feel grateful that both worlds have so much to offer. The clinical world invites us to engage our inner healer. The indigenous world asks that we listen carefully for a call. These concepts are different—and the same.

When clients come to me to prepare for the psychedelic healing journey—especially when they don't have a clear call to a specific medicine—we take the time to discern the options available. We wait until there is enough clarity to make a conscious choice and commitment to walk through a portal that will change life as we know it.

JOURNAL PROMPTS AND REFLECTIONS

» Have you felt a call to a certain psychedelic medicine?

» How did that call come to you?

» Do you have history or experience with this medicine? In your lifetime or your lineage?

» What understanding do you have of how that medicine works? Based on that understanding, reflect and journal on what you feel you need in order to be open to the experience.

6

Intentions vs.
Expectations

*Even after all this time, the sun never
says to the earth, "you owe me.' Look
what happens with a love like that.*

— Hafiz

AFTER DETERMINING THE APPROPRIATE SET AND SETTING and
what medicine to choose, the next questions I invariably hear are: "How
long will this take?" and "How can I know this is really going to work?"
And that's when it's time to begin exploring the relationship between
intentions and expectations. How do they overlap and diverge? What is
an unconscious expectation and how is that different from setting a more
soulful intention.

The current publicity and hype around psychedelics is generating
wildly unrealistic expectations. I've had countless clients come reporting that they've seen the Michael Pollan documentary and are ready to
change their lives. Unfortunately, the expectations they have developed
based on this film or some story they've read is that, in a matter of a
single session or perhaps a series of three, their PTSD or CPTSD will be
obliterated—gone.

I don't mean to suggest that we shouldn't be curious about what the path will look like and how long it may take. Quite the contrary. We should deliberately and intentionally explore these questions, and understand that there is no single right answer. But we must also understand that the length of time it takes to heal is another factor that is informed by many variables—the nature of the trauma experienced, the age at which it began, how persistent or incidental it was, the personality of the individual. Indeed, the same variables that informed decisions about which psychedelic to work with and in what setting also impact the timing of the healing journey itself.

It's true that one medicine session can feel like years of talk therapy. But taken out of context, this statement can be wildly misleading. Imagine that you were to grow five years in size and stature overnight. Most likely, you'd wake up with severe growing pains and be extremely clumsy. This is a good metaphor for how you might feel when emerging from a psychedelic session—awkward, clumsy, and uncomfortable. And that's why it is so important to distinguish our true intentions from our unconscious expectations. There are subtle distinctions between the two that have a monumental impact on the journey and its outcomes.

Changing Focus

Intentions are rooted in curiosity, love, and hope. Expectations, on the other hand, are generally, and often unconsciously, driven by fear or a longing for control. Let me provide an example. A client came to our preparation work several years ago with the intention of finding the courage to leave her husband. While I wanted to support her in feeling some relief in her marriage, I could feel that she was in a desperate, scared place—a mindset that was making it difficult for her to think openly. Despite saying she had to leave the marriage to get her life back, nothing she shared about her partner sounded abusive or unsafe. As she scrambled to explain all the reasons why she had to leave, she often became confused and struggled to articulate what she wanted. I invited her to imagine moving from the place of fear in her body to a space of love and curiosity. If she focused on loving herself rather than fearing all the infinite possibilities of how things might go wrong, how would things shift? How might her intention evolve if she looked through that lens instead?

Over the coming sessions, as she continued to clarify her intentions, much of what came to the surface was how her partnership mirrored the dynamic of her parents. She came to realize that she'd completely stopped pursuing all the things she loved since getting married. Over the last two years, she'd turned to food and alcohol to cope and to numb her feelings. As this deeper subtext came to the forefront, her intention for her healing came into focus. She was beginning to connect to her own agency and identify the unconscious programs and beliefs that were making her feel trapped.

By the time she sat in ceremony three months later, her intention had changed. It was no longer to have the courage to leave her marriage, but rather the desire to release the imprint of dysfunction she'd inherited from her parents. They painted a picture of marriage as a series of power struggles and self-denial. She then set the intention to reconnect to the things that brought her joy.

In ceremony, what came to the surface was an awareness that what felt toxic in her marriage was comprised primarily of things that she had agency to transform in herself. She didn't have to cook dinner every night. She didn't have to be solely responsible for cleaning the house and all other domestically defined chores. She realized that her husband had never asked her for any of this. In fact, he'd even offered to help with the chores, but she'd declined his offer for support many times.

At the crescendo of her session, she opened her eyes and, with tears of relief, said: "I don't think I need a divorce. I just need not to leave myself behind."

YOUR TURN

Can you feel in your body the different energy that comes with having an intention vs. an expectation? If you are exploring healing with psychedelics, consider what your main intentions might be. Explore the difference between things that are rooted in fear or the desire to control, as opposed to things that are rooted in love and hope.

The Power of Curiosity

None of us—even therapists—are immune to blurring the lines between intentions and expectations. The unconscious expectation I brought to the start of my own psychedelic healing journey was the notion that MDMA or psilocybin could cure my eating disorder. My mind had worked with skill and will to forget the things my body held deep inside. The notion that three sessions, even with a psychedelic, could break past the protective barriers of a twenty-year struggle with anorexia and body dysmorphia was painfully unrealistic.

In our first session, my therapist looked at me firmly and said: "I suspect there's something underneath your anorexia. Something deeper that's driving the cruel voice in your head and the behaviors it brings. It's the thing underneath the symptoms that has the most power. Are you willing to consider that the eating disorder is not the enemy, as much as the thing that caused it?"

I was confused and disappointed by her response. Why was I spending all this money and time, taking such great risks (psychedelics were still far from above-ground in 2016), if it wasn't going to cure me? I'd already spent twenty years trying everything else. Now I was barely on the other side of a high-risk pregnancy and emergency C-section, still wanting to admire my body, still experiencing myself as inadequate. It was hard to imagine anything past the immediacy of how flawed I felt in my body.

"Maybe that's the purpose of your eating disorder," my therapist observed. "Maybe it keeps you from imagining anything else. So you're stuck there—frustrated and disempowered. All I'm suggesting is that you move into this psychedelic experience with curiosity rather than an intended outcome. Perhaps with curiosity you will discover that there is far more to your story than anorexia."

Bulls-eye.

JOURNAL PROMPTS AND REFLECTIONS

» Write about the behaviors, habits, or beliefs that you most want to heal and change. How would your life be different without each of these things?

» Reflect on a time when you had an unconscious expectation. How did that go for you?

» If you could revisit that situation now and meet it with intention and curiosity rather than expectation, how would that sound and feel different?

7

Discovering the Inner Healer

The inner healer or Self essence is in everyone.
It can't be damaged. It knows how to heal.

— Richard Schwartz

I WAS HOLDING MY NEWBORN ON THE BACK DECK under the weeping willow tree. The air smelled with the promise of spring. Daffodils sprouted along the wooden fence my husband had built. Everything was as close to perfect as I'd ever known—except I couldn't stop crying.

Somehow it seemed as if I'd found the happy, safe life I'd always wanted. Only I was unraveling inside. Everyone said it was a post-partum reaction. It would pass. But I'd felt this ache for as long as I could remember. I felt painfully broken and undeserving of everything I had. Banging in my head were years of being barraged with messages that if I was selfish or complacent—in other words, not suffering—I would lose everything. I was frozen there, in that anticipatory space, with a looming sense of dread that I might wake one morning and everything I loved would be gone for seemingly no reason at all.

As my husband walked out onto the deck, he saw my tears and sat down beside me, placing his hand gently on my leg. "What can I do?" he asked, looking loving and concerned.

I showed him an article I'd been reading about clinical trials using MDMA to treat people with PTSD. These articles had been popping up repeatedly in my late-night Internet scrolling during breast-feeding sessions. It felt like a sign, a light in the dark—something, somewhere was pulling me toward this path. I was too desperate to question the logic.

"I support you, whatever you decide," my husband said. "Let's find a therapist."

Tough Talk

That was in 2016. The psychedelic movement that is now in full swing was just beginning to gain traction. That was daunting for the part of me that was highly conditioned to comply with expectations and follow rules. Living in Portland, Oregon—one of the most liberal and progressive states at the time—made it easier to navigate, and my husband suggested that I reach out to a mutual friend who might know someone. I called her the next morning, and she invited me for coffee.

I was surprised and relieved to learn that my friend had started psychedelic therapy about a year before. It felt less scary knowing that other intelligent, stable people (who also happened to be moms) were pursuing this path and feeling better. She assured me that there was a robust underground network of therapists, guides, and individuals committed to this therapy. "You'll see," she said. "It's not as taboo as it seems right now. I know a good therapist. She's kind of intimidating, but very skilled." Then she texted me her contact details.

That was really all I needed to hear to take the next step. I contacted the therapist that night before bed. We exchanged a couple of emails and spoke briefly on the phone. She seemed somewhat terse and maybe even a little disinterested in the details of my story, but something about her reserved presentation felt strangely refreshing. We scheduled a preparation session for a week later. It was about a thirty-minute drive to her office, and, as I drove, my mind raced with questions about how this woman had ended up doing what she did and what the process would actually look like.

When she opened the door, I was surprised to find a woman about the same age as my mother—although she couldn't possibly have been more different from her. She looked Bohemian, her hair a mix of blonde and grey. She wore an oversized fleece hoodie and sipped tea and knitted while we talked. She was clearly smart, not just some psuedotherapist doing drugs underground for a steep price, and that was reassuring.

And there was something nurturing about this woman that I could feel despite the exterior she presented, which was much more aloof than any other therapist I'd met. Ordinarily, I think I might have been put off by that, but something about her firm demeanor in this context was reassuring. She'd been a therapist for over forty years, specializing in eating disorders. She had even written a book about her own journey to overcome bulimia. She'd raised two sons and seemed empathetic, but not coddling, to my general plight as a new mom struggling with a history of anorexia. It felt like a good enough place to start and, mostly, just a relief to have found someone so skilled.

"We're going to need to take some time to prepare you for the experience," she began. "The medicine isn't the cure. It just facilitates the process by helping you get to the core of your issues. But much of the work happens before and after the medicinal experience." I told her that I had a baby and hardly enough time to take a shower, so I didn't know how much time I could give her.

"It takes as long as it takes," she said, warning me that I would have to let go of the need to control and measure this experience if it was truly going to work. "If control were the solution to your problems," she observed, "you wouldn't be here. You have a loyal eating disorder that's a master of control. That doesn't seem to be working so well." Then she explained that, for some people, the process took a matter of months; for some, it was a life-long journey. The question was not how long it would take, but rather how much it mattered to me. What would the cost be of *not* doing the work?

I confessed that talking hadn't done me any good up to this point and said I couldn't see that any talking we did in preparation would be any different. I was sick of talking about the past. I thought the point was the medicine—that the medicine was going to make the conversation different somehow.

The therapist was completely unaffected by my resistance. "The medicine does change the conversation," she responded. "And you're going to need to be ready for the world of your subconscious it opens up. You can't 'unknow' what comes to the surface in your psychedelic sessions, even if you want to."

She confirmed that my goal was to cure my anorexia and body dysmorphia, then asked how old I was when that began. "And what about everything that happened before the anorexia?" she followed up. "I suspect there's much more to heal than this. I suspect you're going to need to figure out how this all got started."

What I admired and simultaneously found irritating was her firmness. This woman didn't flinch or tiptoe around the truth. Except for the psychologist who'd threatened to call the cops on my dad, I'd spent most of my life working with therapists who were painfully tender, making me feel as if I were being handled with kid gloves—as if I were so weak I might break. Within two to three sessions, I was usually more worried about them than myself, which was exactly when progress stopped. But this therapist reminded me a little bit of the tough lady who'd stood up to my dad when I was sixteen. I liked that she was almost intimidating. She didn't seem scared of her power or of me, and maybe part of me wanted to be like that—unafraid of what I knew. I could sense that she wasn't going to treat me like a wounded little girl, but rather like the mother I wanted to be. Strong. Direct. Embodied.

YOUR TURN

How challenging is it to imagine yourself as a child? Can you picture the younger version of yourself with empathy? If you are a parent or have children (nieces, nephews, friends) in your life, consider how you view those children and compare it to how you imagine your inner child. What stands out?

Meeting Myself

I've heard the inner healer described as the part inside us that wants to heal and innately knows how to when given the right support. Perhaps my inner healer needed something about this therapist, the chemistry between her spirit and mine. Maybe it was an accident of time. Perhaps it was as simple and hard as finding an embodied maternal presence—someone who was imperfect and was ultimately okay with that. It seemed as if everything had led me to this moment and this experience.

As we proceeded with the preparation process in our next session, the therapist suggested we stop analyzing the past in the same way I had in my conventional therapy and proposed that we shake the process up with an experiment. She asked me to close my eyes and walked me through a meditation, leading me back to my earliest, traceable memory of feeling scared, then invited me to tune in to that memory with each of my five senses. She went through this slowly and deliberately, as if every little detail mattered. What were the sounds? The smells? The taste in my mouth? What could I feel with my hands? What did my eyes see? I'd done so many meditations like that before without getting anywhere, but this time was different.

I found myself inside a memory of sitting on a little mound of dirt, tucked between corn stalks in the garden in back of my childhood home. I could feel the dirt crumbling, sifting through my fingers, like little balls of brown sugar falling back to the ground. The corn stalks, much taller than I was, stood vibrant, alive, and green. They were the perfect shroud for whatever was going on back in the house. A hint of honeysuckle from the barbed-wire fence wafted in the breeze. In a muffled echo, I heard their hollering and carrying on piercing the calm. From all I could tell, they hated each other and struggled to remember me at all. My skin was the darkest, summertime brown, just like my grandpa's. I had on my sneakers and my favorite swimsuit, the one that left stripes I could see on my body even when I took it off. Everything was almost okay out there in the garden—until I had to go back inside.

After describing this scene to my therpaist, she asked how old I thought this little version of me was. "Don't think. Just feel. Tell me the first number that pops in your head."

"Four, maybe five," I responded, surprised to feel tears in my eyes.

"Okay, so here we are. You, meeting this young version of yourself. She's hiding. Can you tune in a little deeper? What's she feeling? Follow your senses. *Don't think; just feel.*"

"She wants to fly," I whispered as my voice cracked. "I hear her praying, asking God for wings. She's mad at them, and maybe mad at God for not giving her wings to escape. The garden is safe, but she has to eat and sleep, which means going back into that dreadful house. There's nothing but chaos and rage in there," I told her, surprised by all the details that emerged.

"I want you to imagine the mom part of you—the mom you've just become," she urged me gently. "The same one who cares so much about her son that she's willing to face anything, even the pain. Imagine that part of you is sitting right next to this little girl. See if she will let you in."

"I hear her humming a little song," I answered. "Maybe she's glad I'm there. She feels so alone, but she's scooted closer now. I can almost feel our bodies brush against one another."

Then this wise lady prompted me to stay in that connection and to let this part of me feel and begin to get to know my maternal self. "It sounds as if she had no secure attachment back then, but you can help her find it now," she said.

JOURNAL PROMPTS AND REFLECTIONS

» Consider one of your earliest memories, particularly one that felt unsafe or confusing.

» Using your imagination, see if you can go back to that memory and connect to the child part of yourself. How can you offer that child a corrective experience now by reparenting her in a different way.

» If you have children, consider moments when they trigger strong emotions inside you. How is their behavior evoking something from your past?

8

Unlocking the Somatic Mystery

*The separation of psychology from the
basic assumptions of biology is purely
artificial, because the human psyche lives
in indissoluble union with the body.*

— Carl Jung

THE WORD "SOMATIC" GETS BANDIED ABOUT A LOT in discussions about therapy. Unfortunately, it is one of those words or concepts that, although used regularly, is often misunderstood. Since understanding somatics and the somatic body is a critical part of psychedelic healing, let's take a moment to define it more precisely here.

In simplest terms, "somatic" refers to anything physical or physiological in the body. Somatic experience is something that is felt physically, not understood intellectually. For example, it is that *felt sense* I had of the little girl version of myself described in the last chapter. Not the idea or concept of her, but the experience of feeling her as real and alive. The body's physiological response may also be to shake or purge, particularly in the psychedelic experience, as the medicine helps us reprocess a traumatic memory.

Trauma has an uncanny way of causing us to get lost in our minds—lost in a perpetual state of hypervigilance, disassociation, or some combination of the two. The net result is that we lose touch with what is really happening in our bodies, in our nervous systems. In so doing, we move farther away from living and deeper into merely surviving. Figuratively speaking, our expression of life becomes an ongoing state of playing dead.

One instinctual response of a wild animal when it perceives a predatory threat is to play dead. Once that threat is gone, the animal may shake violently or spin like a whirling dervish. It may make a primal sound or even attack another animal. Through any of these responses, the animal discharges the internalized stress from its body. But we human animals tend to skip this critical step and get lost in our brains. We shift to a state of self-preservation and remain perpetually on high alert. Rather than discharging the stress, we internalize it. When this happens, we draw the trauma deeper into our psyches, into our cells, even into our DNA.

When initiating a therapeutic process, particularly as we get close to entering the medicinal space, we intentionally talk at length about this somatic part of the experience. To heal, we must return to what the body knows. Like an animal in the wild, we need a primal release, even if we don't realize that's what we're seeking. Often it is the psychedelic medicine that provides the means by which we can get out of our brains and back in touch with our bodies enough to create an opening for this somatic release to occur.

When I arrive at this topic of somatics in preparation, people often start to squirm or drift from the conversation. Eyes gloss over and I know I'm losing them. I know, because I was there for most of my own life—intellectually understanding that my body mattered, but entirely unable to feel anything beneath my skin. It's interesting to note that, for most of my life, I struggled with intermittent bouts of hives—eruptions of itchy, red inflammation that seemingly showed up from out of nowhere on the surface of my skin. In the context of what I know now, all those hives make a lot more sense. My nervous system was holding so much pent up anxiety it was desperate to release that it simply erupted through my skin.

What is your relationship to your body? How in tune are you with your somatic responses to external stimuli? If you spend extensive time lost in your thoughts, when did that start?

Moving Beyond My Brain

I studied somatic therapy and was certified as a yoga instructor in my twenties, hoping that training would help me feel my body. I had recovered from what I thought was the worst of my eating disorder by that point and had cultivated a functional relationship with food. On the surface, it looked as if I had a "normal" life. But what lingered beneath the surface were two problems: control and an absence of desire. My physical body was *entirely numb.*

This was never more obvious than when I met my husband. Although it was the healthiest partnership I'd ever had, my capacity to be intimate with him was painfully limited. My body froze when the topic was broached. I winced sometimes when he touched me. I felt broken and inadequate when this happened, ashamed and confused by my body's response. My somatic reflexes didn't match what my heart felt, and my logical mind couldn't resolve the dissonance. I'd been sexually intimate in relationships that mattered far less to me than this one. So why was my body now shutting down intimately?

As the confusion around this engulfed me, the rigidity of my eating-disorder part reemerged with a vengeance. My behaviors shifted. I recoiled from my partner and began fixating on my weight. Knowing these patterns only end badly, I determined to do the most vulnerable thing I'd ever done. I decided to tell him my shameful secrets—that I was anorexic, that I'd been a beauty queen, and that my sense of sexuality seemed to be stuck somewhere painfully superficial. I felt like a hologram of myself, with absolutely no sense of what was real about my body or my desires. It was becoming painfully evident that the only way for me to relax physically was to drift somewhere far away from my body.

I'd never shared so much about my past with anyone other than therapists. It made me feel way too vulnerable. It had seemed easier until now to feign interest in intimacy, to disassociate from my body, and to play a part. But telling this man more about my history made pretending more challenging. This was terrifying and liberating at the same time. His response of unconditional love felt like salve on my spirit. I still didn't know what to do with my sexuality, but at least I started to think that it might be possible and safe to speak my truth rather than spending the rest of my life running from it.

As I tried to function in the dissonance of what my heart felt and my body didn't, alcohol became a problematic ally. It made disassociating so much easier. I see this pattern now almost daily in my practice—how much we use alcohol to cope with things that would otherwise be too overwhelming. Functional alcoholism is an unaddressed pandemic of our current times. Because a glass of wine (or two or three) is so normalized culturally, we hardly give this behavior a second thought. Yet the disassociation that this kind of numbing creates provides openings for so many additional problems.

Before my psychedelic healing journey, my sexuality felt like a requirement more than a choice. Wine became the elixir needed to make that requirement less scary. What I understand now, after a deep dive through the archives of my own intergenerational trauma, is that I entered sexuality and intimate relationships conditioned by an external and internal patriarchal voice that said my worth as a woman was wrapped up in how pleasing I was to a man. This made the embodied understanding of conscious consent slippery. It led to a significant amount of what I now refer to as *trauma sex*—sex that was not consciously consensual. I had zero concept of what conscious consensual sex was all about, until my psychedelic journey began.

Conscious consent is an important topic, and we will look at it more closely in the next chapter. As a therapist, I find the pervasiveness of this issue both gut-wrenching and somehow humanizing. This is at the core of what the #metoo movement is all about—deconstructing the perfectly curated surface picture in which everything looks fine. Meanwhile, underneath and behind closed doors, there lingers a tremendous amount of dysfunction and a painfully distorted notion of consent. The absence of intimacy and conscious consent overlaid with the heavy presence of trauma sex impacts, not only partnerships, but the children inside those homes as well. It's hard to teach our children a landscape we've not navigated ourselves.

My experience personally and professionally has shown me that the complexity and unconsciousness around sexuality and consent is one of the most critical cultural wounds of our time. A culture that objectifies the body and views sex as a commodity reduces something sacred to a transactional exchange in which everyone exits with less—less agency, less connection, less love. These get replaced with more pain, more hypervigilance, more disassociation, more struggles, more trauma. Intimacy is not intended to be a pantomime performance.

As a girl raised in a purity culture, believe me when I say I had *zero* idea that sex and pleasure were going to become my life's work. Unbeknownst to me, my whole life had been an attempt to escape my body, which held the memory of being touched non-consensually. My anorexia was a brilliant strategy to desexualize myself, to shrink to a size so small that I could feel safe.

The Pleasure Principle

When I arrived at my therapist's office a week after my first MDMA ceremony, she asked me what shifts I'd noticed and how I was doing with integration.

"I'm struggling and frustrated," I told her. "Everything felt clear in the ceremony. I loved myself for what—an hour? Is that how this works? Now what am I supposed to do?!"

"It often gets worse before it gets better," she replied, then told me that, although it seems hard now, it wouldn't stay that way forever. I would have to trust and try to be patient. Then she asked me to tell her anything else I'd noticed, either with my thoughts or my body, no matter how unrelated it seemed. "Everything that emerges now matters," she empahsized.

"Well, now that you mention it, there is one strange thing that happened," I told her, suddenly feeling very self-conscious. I even started to sweat. "I'm not sure what to make of it, but I think I might have had an orgasm for the first time," I told her in a swirl of confusion and maybe with a hint of pride.

This tough lady's face lit up and she seemed ready to jump out of her chair! For someone typically so aloof, this response was notable. She composed herself and leaned toward me as if she really wanted to stress a point. "That's wonderful," she cried. "Don't you see how significant this is? You told me you've never enjoyed sex—*never*. Not even with your husband. Isn't that, right?"

"Well, yes, but that really doesn't feel like the most important issue here," I responded incredulously.

"Do you know how many women come to this space begging to feel their bodies?" she said excitedly. "Some get there and some don't. I'm thrilled for you."

I just sat there for a minute. It hadn't even occurred to me. But suddenly, here on this big fluffy couch, surrounded by cushions, I didn't feel so much like a little girl anymore. It was just the beginning of putting the puzzle together. But in that moment, something I'd never considered before felt strangely clear. Pleasure had been so foreign and forbidden in my life that I ran away from it as fast as I could. As it turned out, the ability to feel my own pleasure was the elusive *aha* I'd been searching for. That orgasm was the end of playing dead, and the beginning of my life.

JOURNAL PROMPTS AND REFLECTIONS

» What is your relationship to your body?

» What is your relationship to pleasure?

» What messages about sexuality were implicit and explicit for you growing up?

» Who talked to you about coming of age? How did that discussion go?

» Reflect on your first sexual experience.

» Reflect on your best somatic experience—the time, the activity, when you felt most alive in your body.

9

Conscious Consent

We have been raised to fear the yes in ourselves.

— Audre Lorde

CONSENT IS DEFINED AS APPROVAL OR AGREEMENT. But it is also defined as permission. How many monumental experiences have you been through for which you were allowed no pause to consider your conscious consent? Who talked to you about sexual consent when you were little? Did that conversation ever happen? How did it go? I knew there was something called the "birds and the bees," but that was as far as I ever got— little rumors overheard while eavesdropping on the school bus.

When my son was born in an emergency C-section, the medical team shoved papers in my hands while I was barely lucid and completely terrified, insisting that I sign "consent forms." No one explained the content of these forms, nor was I able to process what I was consenting to. Rather, my signature came as a response to urgency and pressure, followed by a resignation to comply.

As a trauma therapist, I have lost count of how many women and men have come to me as victims of the absence of conscious dialog about consent. This issue is *everywhere*. And it demands our attention. We see it in hospitals, in cars, in back alleys, and even in our homes. We see and hear of women struggling to discern the nuanced differentiation between coercion and rape. And while we may hear less about it, it is true that men struggle to discern the same distinctions. Women lost in a state of shame, powerlessness, and victimhood. Men equally lost in guilt, confusion, and an internalized sense of being perpetrators. We have evolved—if you can call it that—into a collective state of disassociation and/or hypervigilance. Who is being held accountable? Who is taking responsibility? Who is doing the necessary work of repair? The backdrop of misogyny that lingers strong and insidious in our world will persist until we bring consciousness to it. In the absence of intentional dialog, the patriarchal voice will remain the driving force and dominant narrative.

Epigenetics suggests that these kinds of lineage stories are passed down over time. Internalized and unresolved shame from one generation becomes the burden of the next. The shame threads itself into the ancestral psyche, moving through the bloodlines, weaving the roles of victim and perpetrator like detritus into our generational DNA. The cycle perpetuates itself until someone comes along who is ready, willing, and able to break it.

YOUR TURN

Consider what the notion of conscious consent means to you. Recall examples you've seen of people embodying conscious consent and/or lack of it, then compare your own reaction and response to those examples.

"Yes" and "No"

From deep within the mycelial folds, from the womb of creation, I heard the medicine hum a sacred song.

> How can you say "yes" to anything if you have
> no idea how to say "no?" Stop waiting for
> permission. You're the one you're waiting for.

I let the words sink in, acutely aware that my whole life before this journey was a collision of "yes" and "no." The childhood message etched in my psyche was that I belonged to someone other than myself. My body was a thing to be controlled and contained. If it wasn't, that was going to be a problem and I was going to be in *big* trouble. I learned to let myself be managed, controlled, used, and abused. I offered all my complicity in the name of being a "good girl," a loveable girl, a deserving woman. But where had that left me?

Now inside this earthly womb and deep psychedelic chamber, every scar was revealed to me. Every violation. Every tear. Every other girl in this wound with me. I watched each instance when the female body lingered like a play toy for the misguided masculine. I watched my spirit learn to leave my body behind. I saw how I was groomed for this submission—not a willing surrender, but a predatorially induced resignation.

Now the Earth Mother demanded that I learn to scream the words "yes" and "no." She demanded that I learn the difference between how each felt in my body. She made it clear that I must know this in myself if I wanted to teach it to my children.

The Internalized Perpetrator

Prior to my journey with psychedelics, a voice that echoed my father's wormed its way into my psyche. Many of us have a voice like this—a voice that tells us we are not deserving or good enough, that we need to be pleasing and compliant. This is the voice of the *internalized perpetrator*, and it casts a spell over us as we move out into the world to deal with the battles of everyday life. There we stand, almost as if in a trance, totally susceptible to anything and everything.

I don't remember the specific date when I had my own first failed encounter with the internalized perpetrator. I'd have to do some math to determine the year. I couldn't picture the house, and I certainly don't remember the exact address. But I can tell you how he smelled, the beer thick on his breath and the stink of sweat coming from his pores. I can tell you about the spots on the roof of the car where the lining was beginning to come detached and sag. I can tell you how I pretended those sagging spots were clouds, and how I tried desperately to float away and escape into the clouds.

I can tell you how the next morning, true to Tennessee springtime, the grass was doused with dew and there was a very specific scent of wet hay from the nearby fields. I can tell you how I felt a little bit like a frightened animal, trying to gather my things quickly and get out before the sun came up, before anyone saw me. I can tell you I don't remember how I drove myself home.

I can also tell you I had been drinking. I wasn't drunk, but I wasn't sober either. I was lucid enough to think that going with him to the car might be a bad idea. I can tell you that everything was fine at first. Just two normal, relatively innocent teenagers making out in a car at a party. Not the first to do that and certainly not the last. I can tell you things were moving too fast. I can tell you how something abstractly fun started to feel really scary.

"Slow down. Not yet. Not now. I'm scared," I whispered.

He stopped temporarily. I caught a breath and, for perhaps ten seconds, it seemed as if it was over. But just as the panic started to pass, his hands were everywhere again, faster than I could move to block them. We were back at the same impasse—no longer flirting, but now fighting against each other for power and a kind of connection we didn't even understand. Any intoxication had been scared out of my body, coursed more quickly through my bloodstream by the surge of adrenaline taking over. I was in fight-or-flight mode now, my animal body trying not to die.

I made at least one more attempt at a verbal "no" and, while it was undoubtedly soft and sheepish, it was there.

"Please, I'm not ready."

But my internalized perpetrator was another presence in the car and his was the loudest voice of all. "You've got to give this boy what he wants now that you've come here. You waived your right to say 'no' a long time ago." Then the physical pain of penetration took over and I was gone, gone, gone. I lost a part of me that would not be resuscitated for another twenty-something years.

It's hard to say exactly when or how I gave up my resistance, but there was a moment in which a paralyzing sense of defeat overcame me— a resignation that felt utterly, painfully familiar. The powerlessness of knowing that I couldn't win. It was over in three, maybe five minutes. Misguided kids, fumbling toward adulthood, lost in a lack of support, getting it desperately wrong. How many stories like this does it take to make us wake up to what must change?

I've made the details of this description intentionally graphic. Part of me wants to look the other way, to tell a different story. But the Earth Mother won't let me. I hear her. I hear the medicine. She is still humming the ancient, sacred song. Only now I understand that song lives inside my body. I am the song. When the internalized perpetrator is gone, my body knows both "yes" and "no." In this space, even breath is orgasmic. In this space, we can see that an orgasm is not a thing to covet or sell. It is the mystery from which all life itself blooms and grows. It is not about sex. It is about consent and consciousness. It is the sacred song, the great cosmic vibration. Can you feel it now?

JOURNAL PROMPTS AND REFLECTIONS

» What were the intentional and unintentional messages you received about consent while growing up?

» Who talked to you about sexuality and how did that conversation go?

» How/what do you feel about your earliest sexual exchanges?

» Are there instances in your sexual history when you feel that you or someone you know was denied the ability to consent? How have you dealt with this?

PART II

Ceremony

Everything is ceremony in the
wild garden of childhood.

— Pablo Neruda

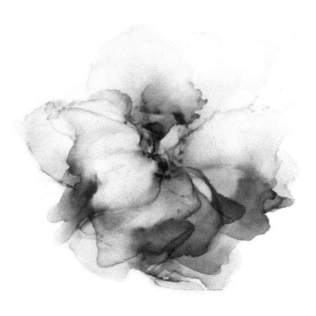

10

The Mythopoetic Language of the Medicine

To be native in a place, we must learn to speak its language.

— Robin Wall Kimmerer

AS WE MOVE INTO THE SECOND PART OF THIS BOOK, we'll begin to discuss the next stage in the psychedelic journey—ceremony. Each chapter contains a story taken directly from the medicinal, ceremonial space. My intention in sharing these deeply intimate, courageous accounts of healing is to make ceremony alive and accessible to you in the realm of your subconscious. My goal is to make the arc of psychedelic therapy less enigmatic for you, but also to acknowledge and honor the ephemeral nature of this work.

Two primary themes are threaded throughout the chapters in Part II—an exploration of the *language the medicine speaks,* and the impact of the *transferential dynamic* between guide and journeyer. By exploring these themes thoroughly, we will illuminate the importance of opening ourselves to a different kind of thinking and knowing—one that exists beyond strategy and logic, one that is much more abstract and interpretive in nature. Moreover, you will learn why this altered state of consciousness is a critical component in repairing attachment trauma. My healing and my practice have shown me that it is the presence of both these elements that makes it possible for the soul to repair from inconceivable wounds.

My personal pilgrimage to heal and the gift of witnessing many individuals in this space has led me to understand trauma, not only as a wound to the body and the mind but also as a wound to the spirit itself. This is part of why psychedelic-assisted therapy is having an impact where other modalities have not. Psychedelics help us tap into the greater mystery of the universe and the potential oneness between all living creatures. They awaken the spirit that has gotten buried under layer upon layer of protective maladaptive strategies to survive. They remind us that it can be safe to live, not just simply to survive.

Now in case you're thinking that this all sounds too esoteric and mystical, let's take a brief look at the science involved that can help you make meaning out of how and why these seemingly metaphysical experiences are possible.

Neurogenesis

The process of *neurogenesis* refers to the brain's capacity to create new neurons and increased neurological activity. This process, which is catalyzed by psychedelics, enables growth, prompts new ideas, and supports developmental shifts. Ultimately, neurogenesis brings forward everything we see occurring naturally in the mind of a child. A child exists (before trauma) in a natural state of wonder, curiosity, playfulness, and connection.

As we age, our minds reduce neurogenetic activity. As this happens, particularly if we have experienced trauma, we feel increasingly rigid and stuck. We want to shift our thinking, but we can't. Part of this is an almost inevitable, natural byproduct of aging and decreased neurological activity. Our brains are done developing, so neurogenesis slows down. However, what science has helped us understand about psychedelic therapy—through clinical trials, data, and research—is that these medicines stimulate neurogenesis in the brain. They make new growth possible at a time when it would otherwise be declining.

Here again, we can see the parallels between what might be understood metaphysically in an indigenous setting and what the data quantifies in science. The future of mental health and the tremendous potential of psychedelic therapy rests in the balance between the wisdom of these two worlds. The more we can find ways to see that shamans and scientists share a common goal—a healthier, happier, safer world—the more these two worlds of wisdom can complement each other rather than colonize or compete.

I know that it's time to transition clients from preparation to ceremony when a palpable sense of secure attachment has been established between them and myself. In the weeks and months we've spent together in numerous sessions preparing for the psychedelic quest, I've come to know their tenderest experiences and parts, as well as their fiercest protectors. If I've played my archetypal, transferential role well, I will have created a solid sense of trust and unconditional acceptance so that they can surrender fully with safety to whatever the medicine brings to the surface.

In the last weeks before ceremony, I give everyone similar homework. I direct them to poets like Mary Oliver, David Whyte, Adrienne Rich, Nikita Gill, and Walt Whitman. I direct them to ancient, sacred texts like the *Tao te Ching*. I suggest that they take inventory of their dreams, as each of these takes them a step closer to learning the language the medicine speaks. These ideas are not new to psychology. Carl Jung pointed our attention toward the concept of archetypes, myths, and dreams decades ago. They couldn't be more relevant in this psychedelic therapeutic space.

Abstraction and Metaphor

When we travel to any new land, it's essential to have a guide, a translator, someone versed in the native tongue. The same is true of the psychedelic journey. Here we require a guide who is fluent in the abstractions and metaphors of this new landscape, and secure in the volatility of unearthed pain. When this translator-guide is there to hold the space and we've familiarized ourselves with the language and terrain of the medicine world, it's possible to repair almost any wound.

I open and close each ceremony with a poem, because this helps clients begin to learn to interpret symbols and metaphors. This is crucial, because that is the language with which the medicine speaks. Psychedelics engage with the spirit and stimulate neurogenesis with a language that transcends everyday interactions. That language, rich in abstraction and metaphor, brings us beyond the literal limitations of cognition and drops us into something much deeper.

YOUR TURN

What preexisting associations do you have with poetry? Do you have a favorite poem? Consider becoming familiar with the works of Joseph Campbell, Carl Jung, and Caroline Myss. Each explores the role of myth and archetypes in our reality, which is another important foundation for psychedelic work.

Poetry has saved my life thousands of times. The medicine found me in the center of a mythopoetic world in which my inner child, my inner healer, and my inner elder lived as one—entirely intact from the trauma. Inside the symbols that the medicine revealed, I watched pain alchemize to purpose. I understood that it was my teacher and my design.

With time, ritual, and support, I came to understand that ceremony was a complete education course on how to live and die. The message from the plant spirit told me to come to ceremony with intention, curiosity, and reverence as often as required until I learned to speak that language like a native. When I came face to face with self-doubt and unworthiness, the voice of the medicine said: "See what I see. Love what I love. It is a long and short journey home to yourself."

The medicine spirit helped me understand that our collective attachment trauma begins with this dichotomy between nature and spirit, between logic and song. The Earth Mother invited me to step into that gap and fill it with love. The instruction was clear. Do not chase after the ephemeral, transcendent psychedelic experience because it is trendy. Come to the journey with an open, humble heart. Come as a student ready to learn and live in service to spreading that wisdom.

JOURNAL PROMPTS AND REFLECTIONS

» Use the following five words in a stream of consciousness reflection: "prayer," "flower," "sky," "water," "time."

» How can you incorporate a practice of giving and receiving into your everyday life? Make observations about how this practice helps you tap into abundance and creativity.

» Print out a copy of your favorite poem. Read it at least once a day. Consider the symbols and metaphors it contains. Write about how some of your favorite metaphors are reflected through nature—for example, leaves falling as a symbol of letting go.

(11)

Your Internal Family System

*Your task is not to seek love, but merely
to seek and find all the barriers within
yourself that you have built against it.*

— Rumi

NOW LET'S TAKE A CLOSER LOOK AT THE INTERNAL WORLD and
the role it plays in psychedelic-assisted therapy. The internal family systems
model mentioned in the introduction comes up often when talking about
psychedelic therapy. In fact, two of the most meaningful trainings I ever
completed in the clinical world explored the space of intersection between
our internal family systems and the application of psychedelic medicine
and what it can reveal about the parts of our selves that have been lost or
suppressed.

According to this therapeutic framework, within each of us there exists
an internal family system that is distinct from our family of origin. As we
grow and face trauma, "parts" of this family emerge to function in protective capacities for the more vulnerable layers underneath. The tender
parts that were most wounded by trauma are exiled—buried beneath our
defensive protectors and managers. The complexity of this internal world

is, in some ways, necessary when we are trapped within abusive dynamics. But it can be hard to shift from a life in which our protectors are in control, even if and when we arrive at safety.

Many people ask how a part that's damaging and destructive can ever be helpful. To answer this question in depth, I recommend therapist Richard Schwartz's book, *No Bad Parts*. In my own experience, the anorexic part within my internal family system was my fiercest protector. Over time, I came to resent this part and the way it negatively impacted my body and self-image. But for me, healing required that I come into a deeper understanding of and even gratitude for how this part attempted to protect me from sexual harm.

This therapeutic model suggests that, in addition to our exiled and protective parts, there is also a part referred to as the *higher self* or *inner healer*. This is the part that wants to heal and even knows intuitively how to go about it. This higher self can be eclipsed by the protective layers and the pain of the exiled parts. When we engage in a healing process with support, however, it becomes possible to unburden ourselves of these parts so that the higher self can re-emerge as the leader in our lives. When this shift happens, we can begin to exist beyond a state of constant alert and self-preservation. We can move past reacting to our wounds and soften into the wisdom reflected through empathy and understanding. This process is not linear. The goal is not to eradicate these parts, but to understand and appreciate the role they play. In so doing, we can offer a corrective "re-parenting" experience.

When we introduce psychedelics into the therapeutic process, they enable us to interact with protective and exiled parts of our selves in a new and transformative way. With the neurogenetic activity the medicines stimulate, it becomes possible to meet our parts with new curiosity and empathy, rather than with judgment and shame. When held in a safe therapeutic container, the parts that re-emerge are able to experience a relational "do-over." Because the psychedelic medicine creates such openness and receptivity, this can be as simple as giving an unconditionally loving response that helps a person step out of years of shame into a world of new possibility. As this happens, the inner landscape begins to change and rearrange itself. And these internal shifts create a safer external reality.

Take a self-inventory. What internal parts are most identifiable to you? Consider your parts in the context of your timeline and index events from chapter 3. See if you can correlate parts to events and begin to put together some of the dynamics of your internal family system.

Finding Maggie

When Maggie and I first met, I could hardly believe all she'd experienced in her life. She was only in her early thirties, but already seemed to have lived multiple lifetimes. Like most clients with CPTSD, Maggie spoke about her experiences with a kind of hard-to-believe detachment. I observed her minimizing the gravity of what she'd been through on multiple occasions, blurring the lines between perception and reality.

No doubt Maggie was resilient. Otherwise, she couldn't have survived. But her need to be strong and survive had inadvertently eclipsed her capacity to acknowledge her own suffering. This made accessing or processing her reservoir of grief almost impossible. As a result, she struggled to stay grounded and described always feeling a looming sense of anxiety. She was reaching for stability and safety in her life, but had no historical context for it, no examples of it, and no blueprint for how to build it.

Maggie belonged to a large Greek family that she described as a mishmash of incredible strength and chaos, of beautiful traditions and deep dysfunction. Her biological father had fled from Canada to Cypress to avoid prosecution as a pedophile, and her childhood and adolescence were punctuated by being passed around between family members, her sense of self being lost somewhere along the way.

Maggie felt loyalty and admiration for all that was good within her lineage, as well as a need to break away from what was toxic. In one of our early preparation sessions, she recalled, as a ten-year-old, finding boxes of pornographic videos produced by her uncle and packaged for distribution. All the messages surrounding her depicted women in roles of servitude and/or objectification. Because her nature was strong, she challenged authority and asked questions no one wanted to face. Because of this, she quickly became the scapegoat in her family.

After failed attempts at living with her uncle and her biological mother, Maggie was sent to live with her paternal grandmother, a tough traditional matriarch. The predominant message from her grandma was that she needed to forgive and forget and get on with her life. Maggie's memories and experiences were gaslit. As a result, she felt distrusting of herself. At around fifteen, when even grandma's house failed her, Maggie moved out on her own, rotating between friends' houses in a survivalist state.

Our paths first crossed during the pandemic. Both of us had begun writing for a virtual community dedicated to the exploration of women and psychedelics. Maggie was looking for a therapist to support her in working through some of the elements of her past with MDMA. We spent several sessions in preparation, building trust with her "council of parts." Maggie suspected she'd experienced things that were sexually inappropriate as a child, but she had no direct memories beyond the constant presence of pornography and the accusations against her father for his inappropriate behavior with her siblings. We discussed the part of her who had never been mothered, who longed for maternal nurture and disliked the vulnerability that longing created.

By the time we scheduled Maggie's first medicine session, I had a solid sense of her main protectors and at least one or two of her tenderest exiles. We'd worked with patience and intention to create a sense of trust and safety in the relational dynamic. When Maggie began to feel the medicine, she got very quiet. I noticed her body position shift and she curled into a little ball. When she began to speak again, her voice sounded younger and frightened. She was insistent on making sure no one was anywhere around who could hear what she needed to say. After confirming that it was just the two of us, Maggie proceeded to tell me about an intrusive memory from childhood. "I've seen this memory a million times," she said. "But I've never told anyone. It makes me feel very ashamed."

I assured her that she was safe and that, no matter what came up, I was there to support, not judge her. I didn't pressure her to tell me anything; I just listened.

Maggie began crying, and I could see the little girl inside her shining through. We'd spent so much time in preparation—working with her internal family system, meeting parts, and understanding the burdens they carried—that she knew how to guide herself deeper into the memory.

"This little part is four or five," she said through tears. "She's so small and she's in the shower with my brother, and I think we're just showering at first and then we sort of touched each other's bodies. Then my mom came in and started screaming at us for being perverted. Oh my God, I can't believe we did that."

Maggie's brother was only one year older than she was. I told her that it was quite normal for kids around that age to begin to feel sensation in private areas of their bodies. I asked her if it would be okay if I offered some corrective re-parenting perspective to this little part who was feeling such profound shame. She nodded her assent, covering her face with her hands.

"What if your mom had come into the bathroom and seen you two, but instead of yelling at you, she had simply re-directed you?"

Maggie asked what I meant, her eyes searching for understanding, as if her life depended on seeing a different ending to this story.

"What if she had said something like this: 'Ok you two, I'm glad you're curious. But I also need you to understand that bodies are really special, and we don't let other people touch us—even our brothers and sisters. You're not in trouble, but it's my job as a mom to help you understand how to honor your body and keep it safe.'"

Maggie asked me in utter disbelief: "You mean you don't think we were perverted, sick kids? My whole life I've been running from that naughty little girl in the shower. I've been so ashamed of her," she admitted through heavy tears.

I told her that I didn't think she was a naughty little girl at all. I thought she was a normal kid surrounded by lots of sexual content and coming into a natural awakening of her body. I assured her, with the deepest conviction

I could convey, that it's not kids' curiosity that's the problem; it's the messaging and the support they do or don't get that causes issues.

"So, you're *really not* disgusted by me?" she asked, as if it were almost impossible to believe.

"I'm not disgusted at all," I replied. "I'm so glad you felt safe enough to tell me so we can give this little girl a new chance and a better perspective on herself and her body." Then I asked her what she thought this little part would like to do or feel now that she was putting the shame away.

Maggie sat quietly, calmly, for a long time before answering. "I feel forgiveness for myself. I might even feel calm instead of anxious. I think I could be curious again, and maybe I can even stop hating my body. It could be a whole new life." And a soft smile peeked out from beneath her tears.

JOURNAL PROMPTS AND REFLECTIONS

» Go back and spend time getting to know each of the parts in the inventory you created earlier. Notice where you feel each part most in your body and what it feels like.

» Explore what each part might want you to know about you.

» Ask your parts how old they are and how old they think you are. Remember, this isn't a cognitive exercise. Go with the first number that pops into your mind.

» Ask your parts if they can be unburdened. What energy or energies would they like to bring to fill the space instead?

12

The Parentification Wound

Children swim in their parents'
unconscious like fish in the sea.

— Gabor Maté

PARENTIFICATION OCCURS when parents look to their children for emotional and/or parental support rather than providing it. This reversal of roles creates a cascade of problems for the child depending on the age at which it begins and its scope. At the root of the parentification wound is the burden of feeling responsible for your parent's happiness or stability in any way.

In some cases of parentification, the oldest sibling is made to be an emotional caretaker for younger brothers and sisters. Sometimes it is expressed as the child managing the parents' relationship in some way. It can unfold when an unhappy parent confides to a child about marital problems, or as a child attempting to be as perfect as possible to maintain peace amid the dysfunction. However it begins, the child assumes too much emotional burden and is thrust into a role of strategy and management. This disruption to normal development of a child's nervous system reflects itself in emotional dysregulation, and often manifests as "mysterious" physical symptoms that are a byproduct of the child's physical attempt to process stress.

The impact of parentification doesn't stop in childhood or adolescence. It permeates our adulthood in relationships, presenting as a need to take care of and manage everyone else's emotions. Caretaking becomes so engrained that most children raised in parentified homes have limited or no awareness of their own needs. Rather they work with vigilance to anticipate and micromanage the needs of those around them. This can result in deeply codependent trauma bonds and cycles. It can also lead to chronic-compulsive behaviors or disorders of various kinds.

Unfortunately, this displacement of the parent's fulfilment onto the shoulders of the child is painfully common. Love and enmeshment are far from the same, but often get interchanged. No child can complete a parent, any more than one partner can complete another.

As a child, I watched my mother deny her desires, dull her potential, and cover the truth of her rage with pretty décor and dresses, all while internalizing a message that ran something like this: *This is what women do—everything for nothing.* My father praised her self-deprecation. His expansion was a byproduct of her denial. Theirs was a dance in which both lost sovereignty, and the child in me was lost in that circus show of hollow symbols.

Family Circus

We had a fire in our house when I was six or seven. It engulfed the whole kitchen before my parents even noticed. They were so busy screaming at each other that no one saw the grease splatter from the stove to the cabinets. It doesn't take long for a whole room to turn to ash, and for a whole marriage and a child's innocence to burn up with it. Most amazing was how they picked up the fight right where they had left off the minute the flames were out. There wasn't even a pause to consider repair. My dad just looked at me and said: "You didn't need those damn French Fries anyway."

When I recalled this event in the psychedelic space, it was like time travel, like stepping from a linear world of right and wrong into a free-fall of possibility. Memories flashed in my mind—my grandpa tossing me into his fluffy old feather bed; a distant notion of secure attachment; a knowing somewhere in my body what safe touch felt like. Then the ease gave way to discomfort, an unsettled-ness inside myself. The surroundings remained soft, but I heard the echoes of dissonance. I saw my parents appear. They were themselves, and also not themselves. I was myself, and also becoming something different.

As this scene in my psyche unfolded, my parents morphed into clowns—circus-like, chaotic and absurd. Their dynamic felt like slapstick, too extreme to be taken seriously. I watched them make messes all over the place, taking perfectly good enough and reducing it to nothing.

I saw this aspect of them in this psychedelic space more clearly than I'd ever seen it before. I was the adult—composed and self-reliant, working so hard to make them feel better about themselves. But all the while, I was losing myself. There wasn't space for anything but this burden of responsibility. Somebody had to keep things steady so they didn't burn the whole house down.

For decades, I tried to get them to see—to see themselves, to see everything they were missing. But in this circus scene, I finally understood that *they couldn't see*. They were blinded by their own misguided ambitions and insecurities. They couldn't see it back then, and they couldn't see it now.

I realized in that moment that they might never see. I also understood that all my attempts to make things better had not really worked. If anything, my efforts had made it more tolerable for them to stay together because they let me manage repair. But something about experiencing this in the psychedelic space felt more liberating than tragic, as if I could finally walk away and know that I had done my best and that it wasn't my fault or my responsibility. In this awareness, I healed my own parentification wound and shifted out of their shadows toward some emerging light.

Dreaming of Motherhood

My life's purpose of healing the epigenetics of trauma plays out most clearly in the role of mother—whether with my own children or in the transferential, psychedelic space of archetypal mother with my clients. Much of my trauma began the moment the child in me attempted to take responsibility for my parents' happiness. Healing has required that I understand that I am not here to heal my parents. Nor am I here to heal my children or my clients. Someone told me long ago: "We don't get to choose our children's karma." To be *mother* is simply to hold a container of safety and trust in which children of all ages feel free and supported enough to trust themselves.

Despite my analytical tendencies and a strong need to control, a core part of me has always been driven by the poetic ineffable. This may be due in large part to the circus scene of my childhood described above. For me, dreams and imagination were an essential refuge from the trauma and the drama. My subconscious and my creativity provided me with a map that threaded through the tumult of my childhood. My intuition wove through my nights in colorful, vivid dreams that were a secret world all to myself.

Given my childhood, I was never a girl who dreamed of growing up and having babies. I dreamed of being free. For years, I didn't trust myself enough even to consider taking on the role of mother. But as I grew older and the window of time to have a baby narrowed, I felt a growing sense that life without children might be tinged with regret. I wasn't sure what to do with those irreconcilable feelings, until children started showing up in my dreams. Not just any children—*my children.*

I suppose it was my deeply embedded connection to my dreamworld that made me take it as a sign when my oldest son appeared like an apparition in my sleep. Somehow, that dream served as a catalyst to move forward into motherhood, despite fear.

"I've been watching you," he said. "I'm coming to help you finish what you started. I want you to be my mommy."

There was something immediately familiar and yet foreign about this dream child—as if my soul had always known him, but my mind was meeting him for the first time. My mind's initial translation of his promise to "help me" was filtered through the lens of my own parentification wound. But it unfolded in ways that were the direct opposite of what I expected and, in fact, gave me exactly what I needed. I imagined that being his mother would make me whole and happy. This was before I fully understood the unconscious burden that places on a child. This was before I realized that was exactly what had happened to me.

Before my son was born, I imagined my dynamic with him as being like a flawless fairytale. I had no concept yet of love that was built around what is real, around consciousness. I had no sense of what it meant for a child to be safe and embodied. This was something I'd never experienced myself. Yet now, I needed to create that dynamic and safety for another. It was an entirely new landscape to navigate and a steep learning curve to climb.

In the earliest days of motherhood, lost in a vortex of post-partum malaise, I struggled to reconcile the disparity between a crushing love I'd never experienced and a sense of resentment I couldn't understand. As I sought in my therapeutic journey to understand all this complexity, I kept finding myself inside the circus scene of my childhood. This is when I started to realize that I hadn't actually had a childhood—at least not in the purest sense. By the time I became a mother, I was thirty-six and had already been emotionally responsible most of my life. I was exhausted and stunted at the same time. I had an inner child begging for a mom and an inner woman weary from never having been a child. These two parts struggled inside me.

Now, in addition to my own inner struggle, I had a baby to raise and no clue how to do it. The maiden me and her naive romantic sensibilities left off where the fairytale ended and reality sank in. With my toes dipping into motherhood, I was beginning to understand my dream about my son in a whole new light. He was helping me by demanding that I tear down the trauma and write a new story.

The original imprint that I had of the role of mother was one of disempowerment. I saw a woman working to rescue everyone without saving herself. This wounded maiden got lost in that endeavor. Then, unconsciously, unintentionally, she projected her needs and expectations onto me. All of this happened in the name of love and in an attempt to compensate for an unnamable emptiness. For me, healing in the psychedelic space and stepping into the sacred expression of motherhood has required that I reclaim my body, my voice, and my agency—everything my mother's generation denied themselves.

JOURNAL PROMPTS AND REFLECTIONS

» In what ways were you parentified as a child?

» Reflect on the emotional maturity (or lack thereof) of your parents. How did that inform your behavior? In what ways can you now recognize your younger self caring for them?

» How do you see these parentification patterns playing out in your current relationships?

13

Transference

*Trauma is not what happens to us, but what we
hold inside in the absence of an empathic witness.*

— Peter Levine

TRANSFERENCE IS AN ESSENTIAL DYNAMIC to understand, particularly within the world of psychedelic therapy. In everyday life, we may confuse transference with projection, but there are subtle, yet significant, distinctions to understand between the two. Projection is problematic in that it often occurs with the people in our lives—our friends or our partners, for example. The challenge is that, despite loving us, even our dearest friends and partners don't have the capacity to hold these projections without taking them personally. Our hurt becomes their hurt. We get stuck in misunderstanding and recycled pain and patterns from the past.

By contrast, in a transferential space, where therapists are trauma-trained, they can hold whatever pain from the past their clients are carrying forward with neutrality, enabling them to rewrite the script of some of their most painful memories and limiting beliefs. In the clinical space, this dynamic occurs when unresolved fears and trauma of the past spill into the therapeutic relationship in search of a corrective experience. Given the increased neurogenetic activity stimulated by the psychedelic medicine, that revised experience—that new script—can then be absorbed into the core autonomic nervous system itself and we can begin to reconsolidate our sense of self around this new perspective.

Alex's Journey

I first met Alex, a trauma therapist with thirty years experience, online. She recounted her story of early childhood abandonment and abuse with notable stoicism. Her intellectual understanding was clinically impeccable. Yet her capacity to feel emotion connected to her experience was anaesthetized. "I am numb," she said with palpable frustration.

By the time we met, Alex had already tried psychedelics, without success. She had seen a shaman and tried taking psilocybin on her own with no effect. Despite being highly disciplined and a strict rule-follower, Alex's urgency to heal sent her scouring the underground network for psychedelic resources and support. She'd read the books. She'd seen the documentaries. Now she had countless clients in her office each week reporting life-changing experiences on magic mushrooms. By the time our paths crossed, she was more upset by her perceived brokenness around not being able to have a psychedelic experience than she was about decades of unresolved, complex trauma.

As I've said before, the desperate hope to feel different is real and urgent, and it leads many to fall prey to the harmful and misleading mythology about the "magical cure" of psychedelic-assisted therapy. Self-defined shamans and guides without substantial training or credentials often charge exorbitant prices for services that ultimately do more harm than good, potentially re-traumatizing the unwary. As we saw in part I, these therapies are useless at best, and harmful at worst, without adequate preparation before and careful integration after the experience. While sometimes people get lucky and have good experiences, there is real danger in using these powerful tools in a deeply altered state of consciousness. There's as much chance of something going wrong as there is of healing.

Alex, like many, entered the experience—through no fault of her own—without adequate information or transparency or accounting of what to expect. None of the movies she'd seen gave a clear picture of how to prepare or support herself throughout such an intensive process. Her nervous system did what any strong nervous system in fight-or-flight mode is more than capable of doing—it blocked or intercepted the absorption of the medicine and the full range of the experience. She froze in the space and walked away feeling worse, not better.

As I listened to Alex tell her story, my heart ached for her. In some ways, I could empathically feel her trauma and disappointment more than she could. Like many survivors of early childhood abandonment, Alex recounted her story as if it were someone else's. She was distracted even though she was physically present. She asked similar questions over and over, but not because she wasn't intelligent. She was one of the most cerebral people I know. Her brain was simply lost in the fog of disassociation.

Given the nature of Alex's childhood, which was characterized by an absent father who medicated with alcohol and a cruel mother who displayed palpable contempt for her children, I knew that substantial preparation work would be of paramount importance for her. If there was going to be any way for her to truly surrender in the psychedelic space, she was going to have to establish some level of trust with me as her guide. She would clearly benefit from a transferential dynamic.

As Alex and I dove into the specifics of her childhood, she struggled increasingly to maintain eye contact. The more I took on the transferential role of mother, the more her repressed fear of her actual mother played out in our shared space. If I was quiet for too long in a session, Alex became preoccupied with the possibility that I was upset with her, that she had done something wrong. She transferred her deepest childhood fears of rejection from her biological mother into the therapeutic container. Then, as a therapist herself, she became upset for doing something she should "know better than to do."

What we understand intellectually as adults is of little use to the wounded child inside. If you've spent time with children, you know that when they are scared or in a tantrum, they do not respond to reason or logic. What they need is to process their feelings safely. Only after the emotion has played itself out can they move into a solution. In Alex's case, the adult-therapist part was repeatedly pressing the inner child to bypass emotions with her logical brain. This is where she was getting tangled every time.

It was essential that Alex trust me if we were to build out a new data set of corrective experiences. My role as the therapist, from a clinical standpoint, was to hold a container of safety and boundaries with the utmost transparency and intention. So I knew that I needed to do everything possible to establish myself as trustworthy, reliable, and safe. Because the nature of Alex's trauma traced back to infancy, we proceeded in baby steps rather than rushing to the medicine. Again, this is because the medicine is not the cure or solution. Rather, it plays an integral part in a complex relational process. Managing the pace and progression of this process while building relational trust was critical for Alex's corrective experience to develop.

After sixteen preparation sessions over four months of intensive work, Alex and I entered her first medicine session. As the medicine began to work its way through her nervous system, her initial response was to ask me to leave the room.

"I don't want you here. I feel too vulnerable. I can't stand you looking at me. Could you just leave, please," she pleaded with visible agitation.

As we've seen, leaving a client alone in an altered state of consciousness is not a safe option. It didn't surprise me that she requested it, however, given her childhood. I knew that, if I left her now, she would very likely experience abandonment all over again. So I suggested that I stay in the room, but not look at her. That way, she remained in relation and securely attached, but wouldn't be over-stimulated by my carefully studying her movements. She would have agency to use her voice without negative consequences. As I proposed this to Alex, all her sensory perceptions intensified, and she reported feeling her heart begin to open.

Alex's desire for me to leave, combined with my need to stay, created a perfect scenario for working through her maternal abandonment wound. The wounded child inside Alex ached from abandonment and longed for secure attachment. The strong adult who'd survived pressed against the potential for corrective connection with fierce autonomy. The adult part, so far, had zero tolerance for vulnerability. These two strong parts reflected in one ecosystem screamed for different things, creating a split inside her.

The challenge was to reconcile the two. Because we'd done extensive preparation work already, Alex had enough agency and trust to at least feel safe telling me that she wanted me to leave. Without the baseline relationship established in preparation, she might simply have endured the experience while feeling miserable and unsafe. As a result, she likely would have walked away with another "failed attempt" at a psychedelic experience.

In this case, however, Alex used her voice, creating an opening for a transferential, relational experience in which her nervous system gathered new data points. She was able to begin to entertain questions that had previously felt forbidden. Could she allow herself to have needs and name them? Could she tolerate a maternal presence who, rather than abandoning her, stayed present, safe, and nonthreatening?

About forty-five minutes after ingesting MDMA, Alex began to have a felt psychedelic experience. She reported things moving and changing in her body. She felt dizziness in her head and saw visions that seemed far away, in the past—snapshots and shards of memories from childhood coming back into focus.

"This is all I've ever wanted," she admitted in a shaky voice. "To be safe, but not alone, to feel my heart open."

YOUR TURN

Consider the best and worst qualities of your parents. Then consider the people who have helped you feel safest.

Going Deeper

In another medicine session nearly a year later, Alex asked if I would sit next to her, which was evidence of how far she'd come in her healing. Relationship now felt safe enough to explore. I could look at her and be close without it being a threat. She wanted us to read a children's book together. This seemingly ordinary parental act was foreign to Alex's inner world. She'd never allowed herself even to consider the normalcy of wanting something so simple and pure. Reading that book in real time together was a corrective experience that was not defined by a grandiose epiphany to explain her pain away. Rather, healing revealed itself in little shivers and shakes through her body, and her capacity to be in proximity with another person.

Trauma does not differentiate linear time. What happened in the distant past, for all practical purposes, is always replaying in the present until we reset our nervous systems. For Alex to move from a place of resisting connection to being open was not a logical shift in her mind, but it indicated an increased capacity to tolerate the feeling of vulnerability in her body. As we sat side by side, she sank deeper into the layers of her subconscious and the felt effects of the medicine. She described a tragic scene of many people together, starving, scared, and unsafe. It wasn't clear initially where this vision originated, however. Was it her memory? Did it belong to someone else?

"Whatever it is, Alex, it is rooted in the past," I told her. "I'm going to stay right here while you process through it to make sure you're safe and supported now. You don't have to talk; just know I'm here with you."

Alex got very quiet. Her body continued to pulse with occasional twitches. After some time had passed, she opened her eyes and said: "I saw my ancestors. It was the Holocaust. So many children lost their mothers. It's an intergenerational thread of maternal abandonment," she whispered in a voice that sounded both wise and childlike.

This gives us a window into how deep our wounds go. Alex's mother wound was rooted farther back than her own lifetime. Woven into her epigenetics was the imprint of abandonment. The psychedelic medicine, used within a transferential dynamic, helped her move beyond logic and defenses, so that the little child inside her could begin the process of reconsolidating her memories. Reconciliation with her literal mother wasn't the only way for her to find a sense of secure attachment. With the help of the medicine in a transferential dynamic, she was able to find connection and safety in her body.

Most of us regularly and unconsciously project unprocessed emotions and experiences from our past into the present. We do this—whether we are aware of it or not—to heal. While this is ultimately a good thing, elements of these experiences can easily get lost in translation, particularly when we're not conscious of what is happening. As you step into the psychedelic space, where the subconscious layers are more deeply accessible, you must be aware of this transferential dynamic and what kinds of wounds the inner child may be working to repair. It's critical to talk with your therapist and to reflect on your own about how to manage this and the vulnerability it creates.

JOURNAL PROMPTS AND REFLECTIONS

» Have you ever been accused of projection? Go back to that scene and consider it through the lens of transference. Now, imagine the projection scenario playing out with someone neutral, offering a different outcome to an old story. What do you feel inside your body as you imagine things unfolding differently?

» What do boundaries mean to you? Are they scary or hard to establish? What would help make them feel safer and more accessible?

14

Pre-Verbal Trauma

All trauma is pre-verbal.

— Bessel van der Kolk

THE PSYCHEDELIC HEALING SPACE reveals that the deepest wounds trace back to pre-verbal experiences and memories, which is part of why "talk therapy" often fails. How do we talk about something that transpired before we had language to speak? Our bodies know, but our minds forget. The solution is wrapped, not in talking, but in *feeling* what that child felt. Psychedelic-assisted healing can enable us to go back to the pre-verbal stage and rewrite those experiences. This can be seen as a kind of rebirth, as was clearly illustrated in the sessions I held with my client, Meredith.

Meredith's Story

Meredith received my contact information through a mutual friend in her Al-Anon group. She sent me a lengthy email explaining a long history of struggles with an eating disorder and addiction, as well as a series of toxic relationships. She felt stuck in her body and her life, despite having tried every possible therapy she could think of. She was adamant about moving forward with plant medicines, and claimed that everything inside her was telling her that this was the only answer that could work for her. It was the only thing she hadn't tried.

Given that I too (as well as many clients) have healed and made seemingly impossible strides in recovering from eating disorders with plant medicines, I was cautiously optimistic for her. It was clear in our initial consult that she had already done extensive personal work and had tremendous self-awareness. We talked about what the psychedelic therapy process might look like tailored to her needs, and agreed to embark on the preparation process together.

Diving into preparation requires a careful assessment of a client's mental and physical health. As Meredith and I explored her story and her past, I was struck by how frozen she seemed. She was deeply empathic, present, and clear. Yet, at the same time, she seemed almost entirely absent. When she spoke about harrowing grief and loss, she seemed totally devoid of emotion.

When clients present with extreme vigilance or disassociation, it's essential to assess more and not simply rush to the medicine space as the cure. In the complex world of trauma, it can be hard to know how much of what a person is struggling with is rooted in physiology and how much is purely psychological, because the body and the psyche are so intertwined. When we investigate cases of autoimmune disease and dysfunction and start digging into personal history—guess what we almost always find? *Trauma.*

Because Meredith had a history of an eating disorder and admitted she struggled to gain weight, it was essential to get some basic lab work done to ensure, from a physiological standpoint, that there were no contraindications for her to proceed. This pause can sometimes seem frustrating to those who are eager to feel better. In a time when people are chasing the ephemeral—and many practitioners are happy to profit from that vulnerability—the need to be thorough to ensure safety and a person's willingness to trust in that is gravely important.

Meredith met my suggestion to move forward in a measured way without any resistance, although she told me she had had tests done many times and that her bloodwork showed her to be healthy. She had spent much of her career working in healthcare, so she understood the need for caution better than most. But she knew something was off. "I don't sleep well. My digestion is a mess and I'm constantly on alert," she complained. So we continued working on preparation while we waited for her lab results. And Meredith was right. Her labs all returned "normal." There was nothing contra-indicating her proceeding with psychedelic therapy.

Most of my clients come to me in activated states of disassociation and/or hypervigilance. But Meredith's disassociation wasn't what made her case seem striking. It was the extreme nature of the disassociation and the desperation around retrieving her memories that struck me as different. Urgency is often a trauma response that needs to be met with a measured approach. Meredith wanted to be measured. She repeatedly told me that she didn't want to force anything, and she wanted to honor the process. She was also insistent that she was experiencing an inaccessible block.

Since travel wasn't feasible for Meredith at that time for several reasons, I suggested that we work virtually. But whenever I work with someone virtually, I insist on an additional safety protocol that requires the physical presence of someone who can give support if needed. This was the only recommendation Meredith resisted. But I knew it was critical for her to have another person with her. That person didn't have to stay in the room the whole time. I would be her therapist and primary support, but we still needed to have someone there for safety's sake. I wanted her to have voice and agency in her healing process, but I needed to honor and hold the integrity for a safe set and setting. Meredith consented to this plan after we explored it carefully.

After much discussion about who would be best to join us in person, Meredith settled on a friend from Al-Anon—someone we both knew and who had extensive experience supporting people with grief. That woman happened to be a mother of seven and a grandma of many. She is an embodiment of the safe maternal archetype, which, as it turns out, is exactly what Meredith needed. Between my support navigating the psychological layers and the physical presence of her friend, Meredith was able to get precisely to the block she'd described.

Remembrance of Things Past

While Meredith had recounted her life story in numerous emails and online sessions, because there was such strong disassociation around her emotions and her memories were so distorted, it was genuinely hard to read how things had impacted her. It wasn't clear until the medicine experience at what age and stage of development the wounding had occurred. I knew that she had lost a baby brother when she was roughly three, but the details were foggy. Initially, she had reported his passing as if she hardly remembered it, saying: "He was there, and he was gone. I never understood, and no one ever discussed it."

Research suggests that narrative memory typically begins anywhere between three and four years of age, so Meredith was in that developmental window when her brother passed. We also know that trauma distorts time and memory. I wasn't sure until we arrived in the medicine space how much of that loss she actually remembered or had experienced. But it became crystal clear incredibly fast as the medicine took effect.

After she ingested psilocybin, I walked Meredith through a meditation, something like the *savasana* portion of a yoga class. This helped her land in her somatic body with her breath and her intentions controlled, and positively redirected her thoughts away from anticipation. Each body metabolizes differently, but most people begin to feel the medicine within thirty to forty minutes. Yet within fifteen minutes, Meredith reported that she felt the room and herself beginning to change. Almost immediately, her voice shifted to that of a child and she began to weep inconsolably. She cried out repeatedly for her mommy, her daddy, and her brother.

"Where did everybody go?" she asked in a little girl voice. "Why did they all leave me? What did I do wrong?"

It was a beautiful and gut-wrenching display of the medicine's capacity to help us get past the amygdala's fight-or-flight system to the core of our primordial pain. We talk extensively about inner-child work in the therapeutic world. But in this medicinal space, Meredith *was* the inner child. She wasn't thinking about anything. She was *feeling* everything. She was three years old all over again. Everything about her affect reflected that—the intonation of her voice, the limited language she used, and the terror of abandonment she described. Meredith didn't have grandiose insights in her ceremony. Rather, she went back to the actual moment of her brother's death and released the stored trauma and grief from her body. I watched her work through the fears, the pain, and the sadness that had been bottled up for over forty-five years.

Meredith's thin frame crumpled as she sobbed, making her look even more like a little girl. As she sat there begging for her mommy, she collapsed into her friend's chest, where she lay for the next several hours. We gave her a teddy bear from childhood, covered her with a blanket, and assured her that we would not leave her and that we loved and supported her. I told her how sorry I was that she had been carrying this weight and pain all these years.

"You mean it's not my fault?" she cried repeatedly. "You don't blame me?"

We replayed the scene countless times, consistently reassuring her nervous system that none of this was her fault. We let her know that she was not alone anymore, that she could stop feeling responsible for everything.

As Meredith began to emerge from the first wave of grief, she sat upright and, with tears streaming down her cheeks, suddenly said: "I can feel him here, my baby brother. It's his presence, his voice. He's telling me to move on with my life. He doesn't want this suffering anymore. He's been trying to tell me, but I couldn't hear him till now." Her face looked transformed. Even through the sobbing and grief, there was a lightness about her, a softness that had been absent before.

"I missed him so badly," she told us. "When I was really little—no one knew—I would sneak out of the house and go lie on the place where they put him in the ground. I missed him so much more than I remembered."

Meredith stayed for probably another hour basking in what she described as a salve to her spirit—this felt sense of her brother's essence in the room. She sat quietly with her eyes closed for some time before gradually coming back into relation with us and processing more.

When I asked her to tell me about what she had felt and seen, she described vivid memories of playing with her brother as a baby, the deep tenderness she had felt for him, and the abruptness of the isolation and silence after he died. "We buried him. My father went back to work the next week. My mom went into her bedroom, closed the door, and hardly came out. It was as if they all died at once and little me kind of died, too."

While Meredith had told me of her brother's passing before, it had never been with this level of detail or emotion. It was as if none of the memories she felt in the medicine space had even been accessible before. She'd never shared her experience of bonding with him prior to his passing, or how she'd visited his grave. She had blocked all of it—the good and the bad—and thrown away the key. Now, she returned to her body from the dissociative void for the first time in decades.

In the presence of tremendous loss, her whole family suffered greatly. And in the absence of support, Meredith did what so many children in traumatic situations do. She internalized the responsibility and the blame. She formed a belief that she must be perfect in order not to be abandoned. She must control everything rigidly, with extreme vigilance. The child inside internalized the feeling that, by being herself, she'd caused everyone to wither and die around her. This belief led to a lifetime of control in eating disorders, addictions, and trauma bonds. All Meredith's attempts at relationships were rooted in the same preoccupation with being perfect in order not be abandoned again.

YOUR TURN

What do you know about your in-utero experience? What do you know about your birth? Do you have trouble accessing your memories from childhood?

Science and Magic

In my clinical training, I'd studied pre-verbal trauma repair and healing extensively, but I'd never witnessed it first-hand in quite this way. I feel that this is one of the areas of greatest opportunity within the psychedelic space. The medicinal tools have a unique, unparalleled capacity to navigate into the depths of the subconscious mind, into the places that trauma has anaesthetized. They bring neurogenesis to that space, creating increased elasticity and the potential to reconnect our emotions and behaviors in new ways. This is the place where science and magic meet.

As a mother who experienced a traumatic birth, the loss of a child through miscarriage, and the "vanishing twin" syndrome, I found Meredith's story in some ways more personal to me than most. I could feel the humanity of grief for everyone in her family of origin. Most significantly for this little girl, Meredith, who was left alone in the wake of her parents' loss, I saw her suffering and what that unprocessed grief cost her. For her mother, in a time with far less mental-health support, I felt profound empathy. And for her father, who was conditioned to be stoic as a measure of masculine strength and had to return to work to provide for the family. How much all of them lost. I watched Meredith's courage to face their collective pain bubble out from under the thick layers of disassociation.

In the days following her ceremony, I reflected on how many mothers, fathers, and children get wounded in the aftermath of birth trauma and/ or the loss of a child. When this kind of loss happens to a child so young and the mother is not supported in a cultural context that recognizes the impact of her mental health, that child is almost certain to create an inner world of complexity and control, as Meredith did.

JOURNAL PROMPTS AND REFLECTIONS

» Journal about your first memory of childhood. Often these memories are seemingly random. Explore everything about your memory and see how many little details you can retrieve.

» If you are aware of any trauma surrounding your birth or in your very early childhood, try to tune in to that little child. It's okay if you can't see them or feel them. Scared children are good dissemblers. Let them know that's okay and that you are there for them whenever they feel ready to share anything, good or bad.

» Try to say hello to your inner child in an intentional way every day. Weave this into your daily routine like a ritual. It doesn't have to be a grandiose gesture or process—just a simple acknowledgment that is consistent and clear.

» Watch children's movies. Read children's books. Most children's movies and books are classic tales full of wisdom for the ages. The more you engage that layer of your own curiosity and wonder, the more you will be able to access that part of yourself in the medicine space.

15

The Power of Ritual

*Grief offers a wild alchemy that transmutes
suffering into fertile ground.*

— Frances Weller

IN THE INDIGENOUS WORLD, ritual is the way they call the spirits home. It's how they weave their ancient wisdom into their current world. In indigenous healing traditions and cultures, ritual is the thread that binds ceremony and life together. It braids the individual into the community and the sacred into the ordinary. It is the bridge between nature and spirit. It is essential to the fabric of life.

In Mexico, the *Dia de los Muertos,* the Day of the Dead, is a celebration built around a powerful set of rituals that link us to the ancestors. This is my favorite time of year there. The intensity of the heat wanes and vibrant orange marigold petals adorn the streets, creating a path for the ancestors to follow to find their way to the *ofrenda,* an altar on which photos and cherished items of those who have passed are displayed. Each year on this special night, guided by the marigold petals, the ancestors cross over the bridge and receive offerings, while blessing the faithful with their timeless, abundant love.

Although not indigenous to this land, my family has come to know it and love it as home. My children were babies when we arrived. My youngest child had not yet walked or talked. His first word was *agua*. My children astound me with their adaptability. I marvel as I hear them speak Spanish like natives. I admire their embodiment of what it looks like to exist as "both/and," rather than as "either/or." Everything about being here—the culture, the language, the values, the distance—helps to wash the epigenetic residue from our blood. With reverence and intention, we've studied the cultural rituals and values of our new home so that we can weave them into our lives authentically.

Raising our children outside of the United States was a conscious choice fueled by many variables, not the least of which was an intention to break intergenerational cycles of trauma and give new expression to the patterns within our lineage. Both my partner and I held deep bonds with our grandparents, who had passed before we had children. Creating our own ofrenda for the Dia de los Muertos gave us a beautiful ritual opportunity to draw the spirits of our ancestors into our family's lives in a more tangible way.

As we decorated the ofrenda, I shared my favorite memories of my grandpa with my sons. They giggled as they listened. Stories about how he waited at the door every time I came to visit. How I loved to eat ice cream and sit in his big, squishy lap while we watched the Grand Ole Opry. How he always snuck money into my pockets. I told them he was like a magician with a power of big presence and few words. I told them about his old wrecking yard full of cranes and excavators—and about how he once accidentally cut off his fingers in one of those big machines. I described how the surface of his grafted skin felt in my hand. They listened attentively. Children seem to know intuitively when something matters. We placed his picture in a bright yellow frame on the ofrenda with a can of his favorite soft drink and a glazed donut. It felt perfect to have him there with us. All the people who mattered most together in one place without any looming threats.

I don't think I truly understood the power of ritual—at least not in a somatic, felt-sense way—until that first Dia de los Muertos in Mexico when we built the ofrenda to my grandfather. Two days after decorating it and celebrating with my family, I boarded a plane to complete my training at the Psychedelic Somatic Institute. In addition to my carry-on bag, I brought with me this living sense of love and connection, as well as a desire to deepen my healing and grow.

Grandpa's Magic

I once heard a curandera say that we inherit our genes from our parents and our magic from our grandparents. My grandfather passed away just before my eighteenth birthday. His impact, even beyond death, has remained one of the strongest anchors to my life. The felt sense of his unconditional love juxtaposed against my father's chaos and rage played like a recurring theme through my world.

My grandfather was a quiet man with dark olive, almost black, skin and piercing blue eyes. My aunt said his eyes were the kind that launched ships. I see those eyes looking back at me almost every day when I look at my oldest son. In ceremony once, my grandfather's spirit showed itself like a light shining from inside my son's little body. "This is how spirits bend time," he told me.

An air of mystery and magic circled my grandfather's aura. I was always intrigued by how this gentlest of men spent his days in his wrecking yard using big machines to crush things. Gentleness is the greatest strength. I was always told that no one knew many details about his family history. They'd migrated from Europe and were believed to be of Black Irish descent, but everything else was more or less elusive. Even his birth certificate was missing. Depending on which of his two sisters you asked, he was born in either 1920 or 1921.

My grandfather's death happened suddenly, long before I was ready to let him go. He and my grandmother had come to visit when I was at the peak of my eating disorder. I was participating in the Miss Tennessee Teen beauty pageant. While my parents had never been able to agree on how to raise me, they had managed to reach a consensus about the merits of pageantry as a vehicle for my future. For my father, winning a pageant meant getting a college scholarship. For my mother, trapped in a generation of perpetual maidenhood, having a daughter as a beauty queen would somehow be an affirmation of both of our worth.

I did not win that beauty pageant. But I'm certain losing on that big stage under all the glaring lights made my soul start to rise up. There was something about parading around in a swimsuit and a ball gown in front of all those people that screamed *dis-ease*, even to the seventeen-year-old version of myself. Something about the pressure of having to be pleasing while simultaneously feeling disgusted by the whole damn thing. Something about the breath-constricting dress in bubble-gum pink that made my vice grip on control start to shatter. It was all just a little too much.

I lamented losing that pageant for a long time, thinking that somehow I'd missed my destiny. If only I'd won, my parents would have been happy. If only I'd won, so many things would have been different. I was haunted for a long time by the perception that I had failed on that stage with so many people watching. It took years, lots of therapy, and some strong psychedelics to unravel the conditioning—to begin to understand that *not* winning a pageant of patriarchal design was, in fact, my true destiny. The word pageant is defined as a kind of ceremony. It seems that, for my entire life, I've been making my way to the *right* ceremony, to the one that feels like home.

My grandparents left the day after I lost the beauty pageant. My grandpa hugged me extra tightly that day before he got in the car and pulled out of the driveway—so tightly that it almost hurt. I remember thinking that he knew something I didn't. I remember thinking there was more to that hug than just all his mighty love. Now, I understand. That hug was goodbye.

On the drive home, he struggled with his peripheral vision. Thinking it might be cataracts, he and my grandma went to the doctor, where he learned that he had a tumor on the optical part of his brain. Maybe it was something about the heartache of seeing all the dysfunction in our lives. Maybe the disappointment about how things had turned out altered the physics and metaphysics of his vision. If he couldn't reach us in this dimension, then maybe he could from the next.

We found out about the tumor in November. He died in February, days before my eighteenth birthday. How could I live without this solitary presence of masculine love and protection? He was the only man who could touch me without making me wince.

I gave a reading at his funeral, a poem I had written about him. I can't remember any of the words, and no one thought to keep a copy. But I remember the numbness I felt standing at the podium. I wanted to cry, but nothing was there. All I could feel was the void of his absence, and the glaring absence of any emotionally available adult in the room.

Within months of his passing, we met again after my car crash. That was the beginning of knowing that his death was also part of my destiny. His absence became my initiation into walking with spirits and talking to ghosts. It marked the beginning of my appreciation of the power of ritual.

YOUR TURN

Consider your biggest loss—a person, a pet, an experience. Now consider how or if you grieved that loss. In what way were you supported and/or given space to express your emotions?

Somatic Release

The aim of the psychedelic somatic method is to leverage the application of psychedelic medicine within a relational container to pressurize a somatic release of trauma from the nervous system. Given that I still experienced periods of disassociation even after extensive healing work, I was drawn to this kind of therapy for myself and my clients. I have watched people with trauma repeatedly get stuck in their heads. In this head space, life is reduced to a hamster wheel of mental management in which we remain disconnected from our bodies, our instincts, and our imaginations.

While my healing journey with psychedelics had already been wildly transformative, the persistent complexity of my relationship with physical touch remained an issue for me. I had a much better understanding of where that deep fear originated, but I still jumped when my husband or my kids entered the room too quickly. Sexual intimacy still prompted a roller coaster ride within myself—available at some times, and completely overwhelmed at others. I experienced my creativity and primal essence as vacillating between on and off, accessible and inaccessible. My body held a reservoir of trauma wanting—but not knowing how—to release it. I hoped that using psychedelic medicine with a somatic focus would help me unlock what remained stuck inside.

In the psychedelic somatic process, we hold stillness rather than verbally processing or managing the body's discomfort through movement. We selectively or consciously choose to quiet the mind and inhibit our own attempts to self-soothe. Instead, we allow whatever agitation or discomfort emerges from our nervous system to swell from the inside out. We wait for the body to take over. Rather than analyzing what we're feeling or experiencing it with language or thought, we attempt to focus solely on the body. Through this felt experience, we can come to understand the cycles of activation within our nervous system and somatically release stored trauma from the body.

In my first experience with this therapeutic framework, I dropped deeper into myself as the ketamine and cannabis worked their way through my system. I felt my heart rate rapidly accelerate. Then, intense heat coursed through me—waves of resistance to whatever I was afraid to face. A familiar felt sense of preparing for battle rose to the surface. I could feel how much of my life had been spent like this, ready to fight. I lingered in that hot, accelerated space for some time. I let the physical sensations move through my nervous system without trying to intervene. I tried to do the hardest thing of all—trust my body, rather than strategize in my mind.

Held in safety by the therapist and beyond my own mental management, my nervous system had its own wisdom of how to find relief. Gradually, my body started to move involuntarily. This movement was not attached to anything cognitive. It was a deeper release that began as twitches and progressed into a full-on shake.

After several waves of this somatic releasing, I became very still, almost frozen. I dropped into the core of my deepest unconscious fears. This felt like tumbling through dimensions of dark, black space. There was no gravity, only an endless descent into nothingness. When the free-fall ended, I found myself inside something like an igloo in a great crevasse of the universe. There was nothing alive there. I was barely alive there. I could freeze to death, and no one would know or care. I saw myself as tiny inside this cave, perhaps two or three years old. Here in this freezing cold space was the very worst of what I felt. Harder even than the constant necessity to be poised for battle was the belief that I was incapable of secure attachment. I was terrified of this nothingness that waited on the other side of the fight.

As if I were watching a black-and-white movie on a sheet of ice that stretched into the infinite, everything that mattered seemed to be slipping out of my grasp. I frantically reached into this dark space to grab hold of my family. I felt a terror of losing love. When I couldn't reach anymore, my arms went numb. I surrendered and cried the way I imagine animals cry—messy and full-throated.

As I allowed all of this to unravel from deep within, I recognized a feeling like the one I'd had when I was much younger in the car crash—a feeling of dancing with death, flirting with the possibility that my life might be over. But in this moment, I stopped flirting and let whatever this great crushing fear was totally take over. I surrendered to the darkness inside myself that I'd been trying to escape.

Watching this little version of me tumble through the black hole, I realized that she wasn't scared or fighting. She was creative, wild, and free. She was not alone in the void, but connected to something mightier than the pain and bigger than the father threatening to crush her. I watched her write stories and draw maps that reflected everything from torture to divinity. I'd never seen this part of myself so clearly before. She was lost and found, it turns out, in the great expanse of my own disassociation.

As this awareness unfolded, little green shoots burst through the blocks of ice in which this little me had been hiding and safe all along. I watched the green grow into vines lining the walls of the igloo. I was no longer cold or scared. I was *alive*. I could feel the blood moving through my body. Inside that blood coursed the felt sense of my grandfather's eternal love. I understood that one adult securely attached along the way can change a life. His presence hovered in the air and, just as I began to reach for him, I realized he was already there. He had never really left.

I heard the curandera's words: *We get our magic from our grandparents.* I saw him in his old rocking chair, only now it was positioned in our house, by our ofrenda. My boys were in his squishy lap, and the medicine of true love had stitched us all back together as if not one moment had passed. What remained was secure attachment and the beautiful character of scars. Inside the thickest ice, the deepest darkest embers sparkled like marigolds.

JOURNAL PROMPTS AND REFLECTIONS

» Consider the role of rituals in your healing journey.

» What rituals do you already have? What rituals would you like to create?

» Research different cultural rituals around seasons, nature, birth, and death. What appeals to you? Why? How could you incorporate these rituals into your world authentically?

16

The Magical Mess
of Imperfection

Hope is a function of struggle.

—Brené Brown

EARLY IN MY CAREER, I was blown away by the work of Brené Brown, specifically her book *The Gifts of Imperfection.* In my childhood, imperfections were forbidden. Vulnerability was beyond weakness—it warranted punishment and shame. Messy was not allowed. To be authentic was to be entirely too vulnerable. Life became instead a constant pursuit of achievements, a relentless striving and a resulting sense of never being enough. As I completed courses by Brené Brown and eagerly read all her publications, I continued to find this central theme of embracing our vulnerability and imperfections regardless of how risky or messy that felt—that in fact, to embrace all of our struggles was to be the most courageous of all. Everything about Brown's work struck me as encapsulating the power and potential of psychedelic-assisted therapy.

As I traveled along the path of my own healing journey, embracing the gifts of my imperfection came to me like a mantra. As I moved into integration and began to heal, I realized that I was living inside the post-psychedelic "magical mess" in which all my unearthed trauma swirled around me in search of a new configuration. Could I find the magic in the mess of my imperfect self and this new reality I'd created? Could I hold on to the trust in my intuition that had precipitated this giant leap enough to find sure footing in the now?

Brown's words came into sharp focus for me as I worked with a client named Melanie—a woman with whom I found I had a lot in common.

Melanie's Vulnerability

As I listened to Melanie tell her story in our initial consultation, I saw that there were striking parallels in our lives. Both of us had emerged from the deep South and were conditioned by evangelical values. Both of us were mothers with two young boys. Both of us had built a life around striving and achieving.

Melanie didn't seem stressed from the outside. She presented as calm, charismatic, engaging, and easy to be around. Yet, she reported overwhelming distress and anxiety. She told me she had a supportive partner and two incredible kids. Her family was financially stable enough that she had been able to walk away from a job that she found toxically stressful. "I should be fine now," she observed. "But I'm not. I'm worse. I want to be close to my kids. I want to feel good in my body. But I'm a tangle of knots." Significantly, she said this with almost no emotional affect.

Melanie's description of how she felt was nearly verbatim what I'd said to my partner eight years prior when my psychedelic journey began. As we discussed her next steps online, something about our meeting felt as if I had come full circle, as if I was approaching a cycle of completion. In Melanie's case, I saw an opportunity to lend a hand by helping her to heal using what I had learned myself in my own endeavor to heal similar wounds.

Melanie had strong reservations about the psychedelic process. It went against her cultural conditioning. There was so much stigma still attached to whether this path to healing was acceptable or ethical. I heard words like "penance" and "sin" reverberating alongside her curiosity as she described her situation. She was desperate to feel better, hopeful that this therapy could work. She was impressed by the emerging research, but fearful that it might not be the right path for her. Her greatest fear was of being judged and punished for her choice of how to heal by breaking certain rules.

Despite this internal resistance, however, Melanie knew that things couldn't stay the way they were. She didn't want them to stay the same. She loved her family, but couldn't feel anything but anxiety. "There's no joy, no fun, no laughter in my life," she told me. "Not even sadness—just the void." Like so many of my clients, she was on a cocktail of pharmaceutical medicines to help regulate her anxiety. She was hesitant to stop taking them, even though, despite their promises, they were not alleviating her symptoms. She was still very anxious, and there was a thick veil of numbness keeping her disconnected from what was most important in her life. In the attempt to manage her negative feelings, she had somehow lost access to *all* her feelings—even the good ones.

Melanie was a medical doctor trained through years of study to understand the body; she was intimately familiar with the mechanics of how to keep it well and functioning. Her mother was a nurse, so working in healthcare was a clear factor in her intergenerational story. Yet alongside this professional focus on health was a pervasive presence of anxiety and autoimmune dysfunction. Her mother, who was approaching seventy, was terrified to retire and suffered from at least five autoimmune diseases. Melanie was trained to take care of others, but it was apparent how vastly unsustainable and toxic the environment in which she had been trained was. She reported watching people who came to the hospital to get better, actually get worse—especially the caretakers themselves. Patients returned with new problems that were side-effects of medicines prescribed to suppress their symptoms, generating an accumulated mess of pharmaceuticals and distress.

The majority of Melanie's first psychedelic medicine session consisted of her revisiting the trauma she had experienced while training to be a doctor. During her residency, she had worked seventy to eighty hours a week while pregnant with her first child. Both she and I had come to the idea of motherhood with a vision of natural childbirth as an opportunity to reset our bodies and our lives. She described feeling the healthiest she had ever felt in her life in the months prior to her pregnancy. She was on top of her studies and at the top of her game. Her pregnancy seemed well timed, she said, because she knew that medical school was only going to get harder. Better to have children now than to wait till she got older. "That's what I told myself," she recounted, looking defeated.

But while the pregnancy was planned and the timing intentional, Melanie, like many women, found herself in a sea of competing priorities, having grossly underestimated the physiological impact of pregnancy.

"Suddenly, I was barely making it, but I wasn't alone. Everyone was drowning. Not just me because I was pregnant. Everyone around me was overwhelmed. It was an open secret—in fact, we joked about it—how we were coping using alcohol and meds. It was totally unsustainable," she recalled.

As a general hospitalist in one of the busiest hospitals in a big city, every aspect of her job reflected the essence of what is wrong with modern medicine. There was no opportunity for root-cause analysis. The care she provided was merely a cycle of diagnose, control, move on, repeat. Her job was to alleviate patients' symptoms, then send them home.

"The focus wasn't on holistic health or long-term care at all," she complained. "I would have been laughed at if I had even mentioned something like that. It was all about fixing the problem and sending people home. And if you couldn't fix the problem, you weren't a good doctor. I found myself constantly analyzing my every move, always second-guessing myself or being second-guessed. I felt inadequate every day. And I was pregnant. It was a disaster."

As we got closer to the medicine session and Melanie began to recount her labor and delivery experience, it became abundantly clear how she'd found herself on a couch in Mexico taking mushrooms. The complexity of trauma stored in her body was simply too much, too deep, to unpack in a "normal" environment that demanded toxic productivity and positivity. The catastrophizing and nonsupportive nature of her labor and delivery experience on top of all the preexisting trauma was simply too much to hold. Logic alone was never going to be enough to put the pieces back together.

Melanie firmly rejected the possibility of delivering her child at the hospital where she worked. "Everything about that place made me sick," she explained. She found a different hospital with midwives on staff, but the residual accumulation of stress led to a labor and delivery very different from what she'd envisioned. She endured a harrowing thirty-six hours of grueling labor and medical mishaps at a time when she had been working an average of seventy hours a week. "I barely made it out alive," she recalled. "But then, it was over, and I had to get it together and go back to work. There was no time off in residency. Back then, the notion of 'birth trauma' was considered way out there."

When I suggested to Melanie that maybe this crippling anxiety she was so angry at herself for experiencing was not entirely, or maybe even not at all, her fault—that maybe, just maybe, the system to which she had given more than a decade of her life had failed her—she replied, glassy-eyed and without a hint of emotion: "*Maybe.*"

Melanie went back to work and did what she'd always done. She pressed forward past exhaustion, past emotion, past internal resistance. These behaviors were not only normalized in the culture in which she worked; they were encouraged. She was praised for bouncing back. Praised for sending patients home quickly. Praised for her resilience and admirable stamina.

And then, somehow, amid frenetic pressure and manic workload, Melanie accidentally got pregnant again. She described feeling overwhelmed with rage when she realized it. She screamed at her husband, wondering how they could have let this happen. "I felt as if having another child would kill me," she remembered. "I love my youngest more than anything and I'm so glad we had him. But I really thought I was going to die."

Remarkably, Melanie went through her second pregnancy and delivery with relative ease when compared to her first. When I asked her how, as a medical doctor, she explained this physiological shift, she replied: "Honestly, there's no good scientific answer. I was a wreck emotionally and already had symptoms of autoimmune disease. I think my body was in a suspended survival state, bracing against collapse, trying desperately to make it to a finish line."

The Power of "Maybe"

Collapse came shortly after giving birth to her youngest and returning to work. When the recent pandemic hit the hospital, that was the tipping point. "Something inside me just broke," she said. Even though nothing about it made cognitive sense, Melanie quit her job and walked away from the career she'd spent years training for. "I knew if I stayed there, I'd die," she told me.

At home, without the pressurized environment of the hospital, Melanie hoped to feel relief. But the responsibilities of a home and the intensity of two small boys under five just left her feeling a different kind of dread and panic—a "home version" of chaos that felt more out of control than the hospital variety. At least at the hospital, there had been a process and an agreement about how things were done. Melanie had mastered the hospital process. But the terrain of home and domesticity felt foreign and chaotic to her, and much harder to control.

As we traveled deeper into the specifics of what made the home space so activating for her, Melanie recalled her childhood experience. When she was eight, her parents had separated. Melanie was one of five children, all under the age of thirteen. Forced to return to work, her mom often resorted to leaving them home alone with their older sister in charge.

"She would leave us each with a list of chores and a stern look to be quiet and behave. Then she was gone for hours or days. We got ourselves to bed and ready for school the next morning. Sometimes things got too crazy, and the cops would come when there was too much noise. Maybe that's why I panic when my kids are loud. I'm scared the cops might come."

Melanie stopped herself as soon as she said this. She felt the distinction between the fear of her inner child and the reality of her life now. Maybe—probably—it wasn't very likely that the cops were going to come to her house simply because her kids were noisy. This was her inner child's fear being externalized. And with this realization, we'd identified the root of an old belief and misperception that the behavior of her and her siblings had caused the cops to come. All these years, decades later, her inner child was terrified, bracing herself for the consequences of having a raging, overworked mother who was also in need of support.

Then I suggested that maybe the police didn't come to their house because they were noisy, but because there were five children home all alone. Maybe they came because a neighbor called them out of concern for their safety. Again, after a few moments of glassy-eyed, pensive silence, she replied: "*Maybe.*"

And the whole week of Melanie's immersive retreat follows this pattern—a series of beautiful "maybes" and reframings. Realizations of limiting beliefs released into new possibilities. It was an awakening, a shifting out of the robust machine of her brain, which was hard-wired to diagnose and control, and the beginning of a softer landing into her somatic body and allowing herself to feel.

As Melanie sat immersed in the medicine state, I looked into her eyes and suggested that maybe this anxiety she'd been working so hard to control was a symptom of not allowing herself to feel what's underneath. "The goal is not that you cry," I pointed out. "That's not the definition of healing. But it strikes me that there's a child, turned woman, turned mom who is dealing with a lot of pent-up emotion."

As I said these words, tears began streaming down Melanie's cheeks. She cried a few minutes before saying: "It feels as if I've been holding back a tsunami and now I can start to let go." Then, almost like magic, her tears turned to laughter. She went back through a whole catalog of childhood memories. So many painful moments punctuated by a kind of beautiful, comedic absurdity. "It feels good to laugh and cry," she marveled. "I can see how we were all doing the best we could and where I got lost. I forgot how to feel. I forgot how to laugh and cry. We need to feel."

Of course, this was the key connection Melanie had needed to make. She had to stop bypassing her emotions and her feelings. When I asked her what, in the light of this connection, she could do to feel safe with her noisy little boys and their wild ways, and to create safety for them, she closed her eyes and was quiet for a while. When she opened them, the sun was setting through the window behind her, shining like a halo. Her affect seemed softer, younger, brighter. There was a hint of hope that had been absent before. Hope, rooted in the real, not in anything toxic.

"I want a garden in the front of our house," she said. "I want my hands in the dirt, a boundary of earth between our family and the world outside. I want a simple life, simple enough so I can write a song and sing it to the birds. Now even that feels like a 'maybe,'" she said with a gentle smile on her face.

YOUR TURN

How comfortable are you to go with the flow of your life? Is it easy (or accessible) for you to find beauty outside of your routine? How easily do you navigate transitions?

Choosing New Pathways

As Melanie and I navigated what came up in her medicinal sessions, we talked at length about how these insights might apply to taking care of herself every day. What would she do when faced with old triggers in light of the neurogenesis she'd catalyzed? How would she learn to choose the new neural pathways, tenuous though they might be, instead of the well-worn trauma trail? How would she hold this reframing of her children's embodiment and noisiness as a reflection of their health rather than a cause for concern? How could she continue to see real life through the ceremonial lens, which had recast her mess in the same light as everything that is sacred? The everyday application of changes in perspective is where the deepest healing work takes place. Healing happens when we bring the ephemeral down to Earth.

Psilocybin didn't cure Melanie's anxiety—no more than any other medicines did. But it catalyzed a significant shift and deepened her awareness and self-compassion. As she returned to her life with new insights and increased neuroplasticity, she cultivated a village of care and worked with intention to reinforce the new trails in her mind. With commitment, support, and time, her anxiety continued to recede. Laughter and play filled the gaps where only anxiety had grown before.

JOURNAL PROMPTS AND REFLECTIONS

» Imagine the most chaotic place or space you've ever experienced. Try to find or focus on the comedic elements inside this space.

» Take an inventory of your daily habits and routines. How much of it is about control vs. being rooted in love and curiosity? Can you bring the vibration of ritual and ceremony to the ordinary everyday tasks of life?

» If that feels like a stretch, that's okay. Try simply to imagine a ritual—however small in scale—that you could perform every day. How might that be nurturing and fun?

17

Resetting the Nervous System

The attempt to escape from pain
is what creates more pain.

— Gabor Maté

MY CLINICAL TRAINING STRESSES THE IMPORTANCE of preparation before and integration after any medicine work. Of course, nearly everyone wants to skip ahead to the psychedelic experience. And that makes perfect sense in our culture of immediacy. We want the quick fix. We want the movie version of everything. Including our healing.

Healing is anything but glamorous. Psychedelic medicines and psychedelic therapy have the capacity to help unlock the mysteries both inside and beyond ourselves. But it still takes hard work in order to feel better, even with powerful tools like psilocybin, ketamine, or MDMA. The mind is a mighty muscle. When trauma, particularly early in life, activates the fight-or-flight drive in our autonomic nervous systems, our bodies shift gears. Once this shift has happened, our bodies and brains stay poised to respond to perceived or real threats until there's some significant intervention.

Psychedelic medicines can provide the intervention needed to shift the nervous system temporarily out of fight-or-flight mode and remind the body what it feels like to rest and relax. This is critical, because it is difficult to replicate something of which we don't have a felt experience inside ourselves. Often when clients arrive, their bodies haven't been relaxed for decades. Their bodies have forgotten how to be calm. No amount of talk therapy, or yoga, or even psychedelics is going to make all that disappear, even if it's true that these modalities can help.

Science and research help us understand why psychedelic therapy is proving more effective than other methods we've tried. Although the experience seems ephemeral, we can explain it to some degree, scientifically. Brain scans show that these medicinal tools stimulate new neural pathways and provoke neurogenesis. And this increase in neurological activity can provide a blueprint for renovation. While this exciting potential is where most of the current conversation is focused, however, we can easily forget to acknowledge that this medicinal experience is only one step in a much longer rebuilding process.

Many recent articles and documentaries omit this "hard work" piece of the story—or, at the very least, downplay it. What remains is an unrealistic picture of how "magical" psychedelics are and how they will unlock the great mysteries of life and heal the heart—at lightning speed. But that version of the story leaves a vast chasm between genuine hope and unrealistic expectations, a chasm in which people can get hurt. It is hard enough to endure complex trauma. To then come to the venture of healing with completely unrealistic expectations can make us feel even more broken than before.

These dangers surfaced as I worked with another client, Will.

Rediscovering Will

The first time I met Will, he was in rehab. When we met online, he was visibly agitated and struggling to engage. He was clearly in an active state of fight-or-flight. Our internet connection was choppy, making a difficult conversation even more disjointed. By the time Will found a private space in the rehab center with a strong enough signal for us to talk without breaking up, he was ready to end the conversation.

Will was in a triage state of crisis, which made him both receptive to help and resistant. Receptive because he was desperate not to die, and resistant because some part of him wanted it to be over. Will's girlfriend at the time had found me online as she searched for resources to help him. She was a holistic health practitioner and had some knowledge about the research surrounding psychedelic therapy. Within minutes, it was clear to me that Will's agreement to meet with me was at least partially an attempt to appease her. He wasn't convinced that some magical mushrooms growing in a field would succeed where all the other tools and methods he had tried had failed. But part of him remained curious and hopeful, and that flicker of curiosity kept him engaged.

"I don't know what I'm doing," Will began, looking pale and sullen, as if his life force had been sucked from his body. He didn't meet my gaze as he continued. "I believe in science. I like data and research. I don't know about all this metaphysical stuff. But this is my third time in rehab in less than a year. I've totaled two cars and basically blown up my life. Nothing is working. I keep ending up here and I don't know why. I feel like a failure."

I told him there was a lot of research emerging and that I could point to many articles and documentaries supporting the therapy. "But none of that matters unless you are genuinely open to the possibility that this could work for you," I warned him. "You have to want to do the hard work to heal. And most important, you have to want to do it for yourself, not for anyone else."

With furrowed brow and visible resistance, Will considered what I said, and responded that he didn't want to read the research, because it would just make him compare himself to everyone else. "I have to decide if I'm ready to face my issues or keep blowing up my life. Right now, I'm not sure of anything. I only want out of this place."

Noting the mandala painting on the wall behind him and the faint murmur of Tibetan prayer bowls humming in the background—indications of a healing framework without any true infrastructure to sustain him beyond the confines of the center—I told him that that made sense and suggested that he think it over and reach out to me if he decided to move forward. "If just talking and thinking were going to solve your problems," I told him, "it would already have happened. There's a reason this cycle is so sticky. The question is how to get un-stuck. Most of the time, it's not cognitive. It's about a feeling in the body, not a bypass in the brain.

This conversation happened in early December. In February, I picked Will up at the airport in Mexico. He was adamant that he couldn't talk about his trauma online or in a conventional therapeutic setting. "I've done enough talking," he said. "I need to commit myself to a different path or I'll sabotage my life." We'd had a series of three preparation sessions prior to his arrival.

I had already warned Will that, before we got to anything ephemeral, we had to face what he'd been running from most of his life. We had to unravel all the adaptive—turned maladaptive—coping mechanisms that were keeping him locked in a survivalist state. Even though he didn't want to talk about his trauma, I insisted that he talk about the experience he was embarking on, and what would be required to take care of himself afterward if he wanted to ensure lasting transformation.

I agreed with Will that a meta-analysis of the psychedelic therapy process would do more harm than good. He was already cerebral enough. We needed to strike a balance between laying a solid foundation and turning the process into a head game. Will was high-functioning, incredibly smart, and seemingly in charge of his life. No one "on the outside" would be aware of his secret struggles, which is part of what compounded his misery and the burden he was carrying. He felt he had to maintain that façade at all costs. This resulted in a crushing weight of inauthenticity.

When he considered how to release the façade in order to heal, Will was overwhelmed. It made him want to abort the mission before even beginning. But I knew that without preparation, we'd never succeed. My goal was to support him in finding that middle ground, where his nervous system was oriented to the experience without trying to control the outcome. To expect anyone to walk into something so ephemeral and foreign when they were used to managing and controlling everything would just be unreasonable.

There are many people who have paid extravagant fees and gone to great lengths in search of these ephemeral experiences only to be left feeling unsatisfied, anticlimactic. Either they didn't "feel" anything, or they felt something but had no idea how to apply that experience to their lives. But working intentionally, it's possible to create a tailored process that is unique to the needs of each person's nervous system, and to design an experience that has impact both before and after the psychedelic session(s). This allows the nervous system to surrender during the therapy and re-enter life after it with some level of ease and grace.

Fight Or Flight

The morning of Will's ceremony, he was palpably nervous. "We need to get this started before I convince myself to leave," he said through a forced smile. I walked him through a meditation as we waited for the medicine to take its effect. Within twenty minutes, his legs and arms began to spasm and twitch. His breathing accelerated. It was clear that he was revisiting something viscerally alarming and tapping into trauma stored in his body. I assured him that I was with him and that, whatever came up, he would not be alone; he would be safe.

With eyes closed, Will described a scene in which a man was pointing a gun at him. As he did this, the twitching in his body intensified fiercely, then gradually subsided. We sat together in the stillness as I continued to remind him that he was safe and that I was there, keeping watch. His eyes stayed closed, but his voice began to crack as he allowed himself to recount the rest of the story. In an act of self-defense against someone who'd broken into his home, Will had grabbed the closest thing within reach—a golf club—and struck the intruder over the head.

Will's memory went blank after that detail. The next thing he recalled was the police arriving at his house. That was followed by blurry recollection of a series of days that were punctuated by alcohol, blackouts, and the first in a succession of car accidents. This marked the beginning point of Will sabotaging the rest of his otherwise normal life.

"I think I really hurt him *really, really* badly," Will said, his voice cracking. Although his eyes remained closed, I could see a single tear in the corner of his eye. I told him that I could understand how frightened he must have been and how strong his instinct to survive was. He opened his eyes for a moment, shedding more tears that he quickly wiped away. "I'm so glad it's over," he admitted. "But I feel terrible. I don't want to be a monster."

"You are a *not* a monster," I replied. "You were protecting yourself from someone who was pointing a gun at you. I'm glad you stopped him from using it. But I'm sorry you've carried this around for so long, and I'm glad you feel safe to talk about it now."

Because of the complexity of shame and trauma, and the persistent state of alarm he was in, Will hadn't told anyone this story (apart from the police) until he told it to me. Instead, he kept trying to numb himself from feeling the memories or seeing the flashbacks in his dreams. He drank to pass out, because his natural sleep was haunted by nightmares. He was locked in fight-or-flight mode because of the extremity of impact to his nervous system. The inability to talk about it was compounding the stress and his desire to drink. The vicious cycle just perpetuated itself. He emerged only to find himself there again. Apart from drinking, the only other outlet he had was to work and be productive. He found himself in a residual tug of war between toxic productivity and a desperate attempt to shut down with alcohol.

In the second half of his ceremony, Will experienced a series of gentle counterpoints to the horror of his traumatic memory. It was as if the medicine were helping him to remember the ways he'd known love and safety before this act of violence. He saw images of childhood pets, felt the connection of his brother and his nieces and nephews. His life force pulled out of the pain and redirected toward love. This happened organically, effortlessly. All the struggle to get to this point, to avoid looking at that most terrifying memory, was the very thing that created an opening for the rest of his life to come back into focus.

"So, this means I can just be okay now?" he wondered. "I don't have to try to hide this terrible secret? Now, I can just get on with my life? Is it really that simple?"

"I don't know that it's simple," I replied. "But I think it's a brave and necessary beginning." Noting how much softer his face looked and how calm his energy felt, I asked him if his body felt different now than it had before?

"I feel I can breathe for the first time in over a year," he answered with a huge sigh.

Rest and Digest

Framing expectations after coming out of the psychedelic space is just as important as it is going in. Again, if we think this experience is going to cure us, we're just setting ourselves up for disappointment. Yet this can be so easy to do in that moment in the medicine space when self-empathy is so much more accessible. When we're not in fight-or-flight mode, our bodies feel different and our thoughts change. The challenge is to hold that self-empathy as we return to our lives in the wake of releasing the emotions.

Following an earthquake, there are aftershocks, and this is an apt metaphor for the psychedelic healing process. After the psychedelic experience, our memories and our sense of self is intentionally shaken at the foundation. This is the catalyst to reorganizing our stories and our lives. But it's a starting point, not an end goal. Will and I talked at length about how to take his newfound sense of calm home with him. We discussed the potential for relapse into alcohol abuse, how to avoid it, and how to love himself through it if it happened. We talked about the danger of the stresses and triggers of life and old memories inevitably resuming if he defaulted to the old neural pathways rather than choosing the new ones.

In late March, Will called me unexpectedly without any meeting scheduled on my calendar. I knew when I saw the unexpected call that something had happened. When I answered my phone, it was clear that he was intoxicated. "Don't worry. I'm in a taxi," he said, slurring the words. Then he told me that, that day, he had returned to the house where the violent incident had occurred to get some of his belongings. Being in that space conjured up memories and feelings of shame. When everything flooded back in, he went to the tool he was most familiar with—alcohol—even though he knew it wouldn't work.

"I knew this wasn't the choice anymore," he explained. "I know I'm intoxicated now, but somehow I still feel different. I needed to prove to myself that the alcohol doesn't work anymore. I don't want to die anymore. I want to live."

It's been over a year since that call and Will is still sober without the desire for alcohol to cope. There have been plenty of triggers, but none of them have led to drink. Will's life is dramatically different in multiple ways. He moved to a new house. He rekindled old friendships and built new ones. He stopped hiding from life. His business is growing in a sustainable way and he's learned to give himself permission to have boundaries. He's using his voice to talk authentically about what he's been through.

When I met Will, none of these things would have been possible. The psychedelic process helped him remember his essence beyond the trauma. It reminded him that he was more than the sum of his pain and that, above all else, he is a good human being with a healthy instinct for self-preservation. He continues his path of healing and has grown to see even talk therapy as a useful endeavor. "It all makes sense now that I understand what I really need to talk about," Will told me in one of our most recent sessions.

Will's story is a somewhat extreme example. But in some ways, it isn't. We live in a time punctuated by traumatic experiences and violence—school shootings, sociopolitical turbulence, the prevalence of sexual manipulation and abuse. Our nervous systems are flooded daily with extremely stress-ful stimuli. Yet we are often encouraged, explicitly or implicitly, to press through, to compartmentalize our feelings and get on with life.

We exist in a time when we're conditioned to think that, if we're not literally dying, we must be fine. We're led to believe that the best solutions are the ones that suppress symptoms the fastest. But in fact, most often, the things we're doing to suppress symptoms are just creating more problems. We've normalized unhealthy coping mechanisms like daily alcohol consumption and elevated quick fixes; we praise people for maintaining appearances while dying inside.

While Will's story may have a more dramatic climax than most, the essence of his trauma shares a common theme. He built a life around coping with repressed trauma by pushing himself at a toxic productivity pace. This cycle was leading him nearer each day to self-sabotage and disease. The psychedelic therapy process didn't cure his problems, but it helped him to tolerate the intensity of getting to the root cause. Once at that level, he was able to forgive himself and begin to reconsolidate his sense of self-worth and self-love. He was able to rest and digest.

JOURNAL PROMPTS AND REFLECTIONS

» What memory haunts you? Can you look at it? What happens when you try?

» If that is too overwhelming, don't worry! Try this instead. Consider the bravest person you know, or any heroic characters portrayed in books or movies. How did they face danger or threats? What was it about their behavior that made them heroic?

» Now consider if these characters made mistakes and/or had flaws. In what ways were those flaws also directly or indirectly connected to their strengths.

» Can you see something redeemable in even your darkest hour?

18

Sexual Trauma

*I swore never to be silent whenever and
wherever human beings endure suffering and
humiliation. We must take sides. Neutrality
helps the oppressor, never the victim. Silence
encourages the tormentor, never the tormented.*

— Elie Wiesel

BEFORE TRANSITIONING TO PSYCHEDELIC THERAPY, I spent
more than a decade working as a certified life coach. When I began working as a psychedelic therapist, parts of me felt like an imposter because I
didn't have a clinical degree in psychology. I'd intentionally gone a different
route in my education and professional path. As a student, I began exploring philosophy and psychology. As I studied them both, I found myself
drawn to the former. Philosophy focused more on asking questions than
on analyzing answers. Something about being involved in the questions
resonated with me. It felt more challenging and earnest.

In the third medicine session of my personal healing process, I heard
a firm, but gentle, voice say: "*This* is your calling. Now heal your heart,
because you're going to need to know a lot of things."

Everything got quiet and still.

Then the same voice said: "Trauma is the teacher. Pain is the initiation. Now go. Get to work."

Those words were both exciting and terrifying. I had no shortage of experience supporting people, but this was categorically a different level of support. I knew I needed much more training and healing to be ready to hold psychedelic space, and I spent the next three years working with multiple therapists and mentors. I believed in my capability at the core. But I was also highly skeptical of people who, after one or two ceremonies, decided to call themselves "shamans" or "healers." These are not titles we can simply take on. To be a shaman or a healer in the indigenous world is to be born into that lineage. It is all they have ever known.

The closest thing to such a tradition in my own lineage was the epigenetic imprint of midwifery, which is how I've come to see my role over time. I see this as a great rekindling of the energy of my ancestors who, for many generations, delivered babies in the backwoods of Tennessee. The birth space feels intimately known to me, as if my DNA recognizes it immediately. In this space, where so many things can go wrong, I feel most at home and connected to my intuition.

Tapping into this ancestral trust required more healing work than I could have imagined. I started psychedelic therapy after copious research and declared that I would do three ceremonies according to the clinical model. Then I would be healed and able to get back to the rest of my life. Here I am eight years later—still studying, still healing.

There is no single path that is perfectly designed to prepare you for this work. But it is critical—now more than ever, as legalization rapidly sweeps across the country—that we get clear on what is and is not safe in this space and how to mitigate harm. My experience with Lola demonstrated that to me in a most painful way.

Losing Lola

My first mentor told me that every client who came to me for help would also be my teacher. This was certainly the case with Lola. My experience with her ripped me out of the imposter syndrome into the awakening of responsibility. What I witnessed happen to Lola propelled me into action. She helped me understand that passivity is complicity. And passive was not something I was willing to be.

Lola was a coaching client from years prior. The last time I saw her in person was at a retreat for an organization where I provided professional-development services. Lola was a valued employee of the company at the time. On this particular day, she was especially radiant.

I knew Lola struggled with her mental health and had a history of trauma. Any time her trauma came up, she quickly changed the subject or minimized the impact. This is common among survivors of abuse, as I've noted many times already. Abusers typically deny what happened in hopes that their victims will stop believing themselves. Over time, victims of abuse learn to minimize or deny their memories in order to survive. While this enables them to get through the immediacy of trauma, it becomes a sickening loyalty bond in which it's very easy to get perpetually lost.

Lola and I maintained contact over the years, even when our professional paths took different directions. She reached out periodically when she needed support for making big decisions, but I hadn't spoken to her in quite some time. My psychedelic therapy practice was just starting to grow when I got an unexpected and panicked call from her. She'd made all kinds of seemingly abrupt, significant changes in her life, including ending a relationship with a long-time partner. She spoke at hyper speed, her voice frantic and distressed.

When I asked her if she was okay, Lola told me that she had gone to "a strange retreat" that was the best thing that had ever happened to her. "Or maybe the worst," she added, with her voice cracking. "I'm still trying to figure it out." When I asked what she meant, she fumbled through a tearful reply.

"I took a flyer about plant medicines from my yoga studio," she told me. "I'd been wanting to try it even though it was a lot of money—$3,500. But I needed help and I thought this might be the answer. I've read so many articles about how I could heal myself. At first, the medicine felt amazing—as if my whole life started making sense. Then everything changed abruptly, and that's where it gets foggy."

I prompted her gently for details, and found myself cringing at her reply.

"Well, it was amazing at first. And then the man who was facilitating started to touch my leg. He kept doing it and I wanted to ask him to stop, but I couldn't get my voice to work. I felt so scared, and then I started seeing my dad's face in his face. It was awful. I'm so ashamed and confused." I could feel that she was on the edge of a panic attack, so I told her that I worked with plant medicines and had been trained as a therapist, and said that I would do my best to help her. I apologized for this awful experience she'd had.

We planned to meet every week and I helped her find a naturopath so she could get some basic tests done to evaluate how her body was navigating the stress. Fortunately, she had health coverage through her job, so she was able to access support. But she was utterly stressed about people seeing her in such a state of dysregulation. She continued to push herself as she always did, or perhaps even harder to overcompensate.

She needed a village of care, and seemingly had no one. Her ex-partner was relatively supportive, but her parents had already passed. Her family of origin was a portal to generations of trauma. She had one half-sister who refused to believe any of the things Lola shared. Apart from that, there was no one except a son she'd had when she was very young who was the light of her life.

In our weekly sessions, Lola unpacked the memories of what had happened as much as her internal defenses would allow. The details were fuzzy, but the man facilitating the experience insisted that healing must include "reparative touch." He started with a gentle caress on her feet and legs. By the time he got to her knee, she blacked out. She was never informed of what medicines she'd consumed or in what dosages.

I asked her for the name of the facility and facilitator and tried to call the number she gave me. I left a message saying that I was Lola's therapist and had been authorized to speak on her behalf. No one returned the call. I tried again a couple of days later, and found that the number was out of service. There was no website or any other way that I could track this person down. Lola said there were fifteen participants at the retreat (at $3,500 apiece!), but she only knew one other woman from her yoga class. When Lola reached out to her, she didn't respond.

The pandemic struck just as Lola was starting to stabilize from this horrific experience. With normal outlets and coping mechanisms unavailable, Lola began missing our meetings and sounding increasingly manic—clear red flags. She kept insisting on her need to wash herself over and over, sometimes as many as twenty times a day. "I can't get my body clean enough ever," she said through tears.

About six weeks into the pandemic lockdown, I saw a post on Lola's social media that rang out like a cry for help. She referenced suicidal thoughts and child sexual abuse in a voice that was raw, angry, and alarming. I attempted to reach her repeatedly, but to no avail. The following day, I got a message from the person she'd been living with saying that she had been placed in a mental-health facility, having been diagnosed with bipolar disorder. She was placed on lithium.

Lola called me when she left the facility. We tried to pick up where we had left off, but, at this point, she was oscillating wildly between numbness and hope, punctuated by moments of extreme desperation. She wanted to wean herself off the pharmaceuticals she'd been required to take at the facility, because they just made her feel worse.

The last time we talked, I had a sinking feeling through the entire meeting. She sounded one part manic and the rest visionary. She spoke in grandiose terms and ideas, sharing visions from her dreams, displaying classic symptoms of a psychotic break. She had abruptly stopped taking all her medications. She threatened to "go after" the man who had violated her, then asked: "Why does it seem that people learn more from the hurt and the dark than from being good?" The conversation ended with her thanking me for always listening and for seeing her.

And that was the last time we ever spoke.

We were supposed to meet the following week, but she didn't show up and I was scheduled to travel for work that same day. We'd been in communication two days prior, but a lot can change in two days when you're in a manic episode. My last message from her was a text with a picture of herself and her son at dinner.

"My happy place," it said.

I kept my phone on as long as I could before the plane departed. By the time we landed, I had multiple messages from Lola's roommate. I felt a lump in my throat and nausea in my stomach. I barely made it to the bathroom before vomiting. I hadn't even listened to the voicemails yet, but I knew.

"Lola left us yesterday. She loved you very much. You were one of a small handful of people she trusted. Thank you for being there."

YOUR TURN

Have you lost anyone to suicide and/or mental-health struggles? What do you know and understand about repressed memories? Do you know people who've been given a diagnosis or a medication, and then watched them get worse instead of better?

Hard Lessons

Lola's story taught me in a very painful way how much can go wrong in the psychedelic space. What defines how things unfold is a combination of several critical elements, including the skill, training, and integrity of the guide, and the container in which the work is done. The preparedness of the individual walking into that space, their mindset, is also paramount. And above all, there must be transparency and conscious consent. The vast majority of trauma is wrapped up in the absence of consent. We cannot repair violation without consent. Because the healing journey is hard to define and unpredictable at times, consent must be reaffirmed at every fork in the road. It is not a one-and-done arrangement.

From the first session with clients, I begin a conversation about what it means to consent consciously. Every person I've worked with has come to me, at least in part, to heal from the wound of having their consent ignored. This means that they are still cultivating their voice and their agency to set boundaries. We cannot say "yes" to anything if we cannot first say "no." Consent in the psychedelic space begins with saying "yes" to the understanding that we're embarking on a healing path that will evoke huge emotions and unresolved trauma. We're saying "yes" to understanding that this unearthing can leave us feeling wildly out of control.

Before any deeper healing can happen, we must be entirely aligned in our consent to face that pain. That conscious consent becomes our buoy when the process is most challenging. Many practitioners leap ahead, defining consent in terms of corrective touch or nurture. But touch should only be used miles down the road—*if ever*. Before others can say "yes" or "no" to touch, they must feel safe inside their own skins. The corrective experience begins by being held in relational safety with a trained facilitator who witnesses the client's process without turning away. Being witnessed, not rescued, is the origin of rehabilitation.

Remember that this is not our first psychedelic renaissance. There are too many stories emerging about practitioners in this unsanctioned space saying and doing all sorts of things that are retraumatizing at the least, and soul-crushing at the worst. This was Lola's experience. This is the dark side of psychedelics. And there are already far too many disturbing accounts of when, where, and how this work can go from healing to re-traumatization painfully fast.

Lola is more than a statistic for me. She was a real human being for whom I cared immensely. She was also desperately seeking help. Along that path, she got even more wounded. Her transition out of this life made it impossible for me to sit on the sidelines anymore. Whatever part inside me that still struggled with imposter syndrome crumbled in the aftermath of her death. From that moment, it became my mission to do all I could to make this work accessible and safe.

As I struggled with the tragedy of Lola's departure from this Earth, I sought extensive support. I cried. I yelled. My mentors, colleagues, and friends listened and held space for me. I grieved. I signed up for more trainings. I joined more organizations focused on harm-reduction. I did everything I could think of to stand in opposition to stories like these. I started teaching a class on safety, healing, and transformation, and this book grew out of that class. I committed to Lola's spirit that I would tell her story so that some justice and accountability would follow.

After the intense rawness and grief from Lola's suicide subsided, I took my intention for healing around this wound like a prayer to the medicine space. My intent was to understand how I could be of deeper service. How I could mitigate the likelihood of more stories like what Lola had experienced happening.

Within minutes, I heard Lola's voice—no longer manic, but steady and clear. "I'm free," she said. "Death is a teacher, as is life. I don't feel haunted anymore. My life is not a tragedy, but an insistence for accountability. I am a reminder that there is a fine line between breakdown and breakthrough. Balanced on that tightrope, we can never look away."

Lola's passing awakened my sense of purpose and made me realize the urgent need for increased education, awareness, and access as it pertains to psychedelic therapy. I cannot say it enough. *The potential for harm is as real as the potential for healing.* And it's a fine line to navigate.

Any one of us stepping into psychedelic therapy to hold space for others must remember that the impetus to comfort through touch, while incredibly loaded in general, is particularly dangerous in delicate states of altered consciousness. The impetus to rescue is even more painfully misguided. We are there as guides to invite others to remember their own internal strength—to help them save themselves. We do that by mirroring back their own capacities, not by making ourselves heroes.

People come to psychedelic therapy because nothing they've tried so far has worked. Psilocybin, ketamine, or MDMA are rarely a first attempt at repair. They are most often a last resort, an act of desperation to leave the pain stories behind. Clients in first consultations often make some version of this statement: "I feel as if I'm about 85 percent better, but the rest of me is utterly stuck."

Talking doesn't get us to the root. Somatic work may bring us closer. But if the wounding was connected to the body, as was Lola's case, we might be so disassociated that we can't feel what is there. In a safe container, with proper preparation before and solid integration after, Lola's story might have had a very different ending.

In one of our integration sessions, as Lola attempted to process her experience with the man at the retreat, she told me that what stood out most for her was the repressed memory that surfaced of her father's face. "I could sense in my body that this had happened before. I tried for years to talk to my family about it, but everyone shut it down. No one wanted to look. No one wanted to listen."

This is how intergenerational cycles of abuse persist. The shame makes them intolerable to face. It is our responsibility, now more than ever, not to look away.

JOURNAL PROMPTS AND REFLECTIONS

» Do you have memories that feel present, but foggy—as if you can see them, but have no attachment to them at all, almost like a phantom limb? If so, write about these memories and try to recall as much detail as possible.

» If you have siblings, consider their behavior, their lifestyle. In what ways can you see patterns of dysfunction present in the family system?

» What does consent mean to you?

19

Beyond the Haunting

*If you look deeply into the palm of your hand,
you will see your parents and all generations
of your ancestors. All of them are alive in this
moment. Each is present in your body. You are
the continuation of each of these people.*

— Thich Nhat Hanh

IN THIS CHAPTER, I SHARE HOW THE MEDICINAL TOOLS helped me unpack an intergenerational story of shame. Despite years of analyzing my family of origin in cognitive talk therapy, these insights had never crystalized as they did in the medicine space. By tapping into something more metaphysical and noncognitive, I was able to identify the pervasive secrets that were a source of mental illness and dis-ease in my family system.

Despite my mind's desire to protect me from the most painful memories of my past, those very secrets created deep imbalances and illness within the ecosystem of myself. Once those secrets were released, my body course-corrected with a kind of innate wisdom. Before psychedelic therapy, discerning the wiser voice of my intuition from the survivalist voice of my protective mind was practically impossible.

The defense mechanisms of the traumatized mind can be incredibly rigid and deeply unconscious. But it is critical to remember that this restrictive state of defense and self-preservation is not reflective of a "bad" part inside ourselves. Arguably, it is that instinct to survive and all the adaptive strategies and parts born from that place that keep us alive in the face of great trauma.

Cautionary Tales

My favorite auntie on my father's side told me to be careful. She said it with a wink, but I knew it was a warning. She was the tough one in the family—feisty and commanding. I admired that in her. I didn't see the other women in my family command authority in the same way. She was bossy and unapologetic, and people listened. When she walked in the door, men and boys scurried like mice. "You don't need to be scared of them boys," she told me with an unfamiliar earnestness. "Girls are stronger; we know things they don't."

Just like that, she turned my world on a dime. She gave a hint of something otherwise forbidden. She gave me permission to know things. She tried to prepare me for the fact that knowing things can be dangerous, but back then we only spoke in whispers and code.

Trauma spreads through my bloodlines like bamboo, strong and supple. Sometimes dressed as madness. Sometimes as addiction. Sometimes as violence. It wears many faces and has many names, but lies hidden with everything that is evocative of shame.

It took years for me to understand that inside everything labeled as trauma there also rests a jewel—a seeing, a knowing, a power. Intuition is the key that unlocks that house of treasure, inside of which there is no battle for control, only truth and clarity. Inside that house, I sleep like a baby and walk like a warrior in tune with the Earth. Inside that house, my life is my own and I understand my life to be a gift, not a curse.

This was the truth revealed to me under the elixir of the great mycelium and her perfect flowering body. How little I understood about this vast network under the soil. All of life held in the womb of nature where she spreads and pulses her rhythms into the world, like a woman in labor. My great-aunties were midwives. They whispered this knowing in my ears through the mycelial womb.

When the psilocybin carried me into the soil, my aunties showed me the intricate weave of my ancestors. In a voice that was familiar, loving, and firm, they insisted that my self-concept deconstruct. They repeated this until it was all I knew. Until my ego completely dissolved, returning me to the Earth and revealing how subservience and humility left little space for agency.

I saw myself inside the construct of time, chasing the truth like an elusive thread. I was the canary in the coal mine of my lineage, holding my karmic inheritance. I'd come to sing a song and not be sorry, where the women before me had predominantly been silenced and shamed.

I saw the vastness of what was buried in the cemetery just behind my grandma's old farmhouse. The garden, fertile and ripe, succulent tomatoes popping off the vine and toppling like offerings onto the graves. Death and life juxtaposed, swirling together in the soil—lushness and loss represented in equal measure.

My cousin commanded the four-wheeler like a master at age eleven while I clung to his waist, pink frock and blonde curls streaming behind. I felt a shiver on my spine as we whizzed past the cemetery where the ghosts grasped my feet. Etched in the family code was reverence to a god who required that we reject our desires and curiosities, who taught that feeling sorry was an inherent part of being alive. I was raised to tell half-truths and leave the rest behind. I learned to subvert my power in an attempt to find a place in a world that was not ever mine.

Fathers and Sons

I never met my paternal grandfather. He was dead before I came along, buried in that cemetery. My grandmother visited him daily, loyal to a man she had loved almost as deeply as she despised him. His stories linger large. He was charismatic and unhinged, prone to episodic drunken outbursts before the war, from which his body returned, but not his spirit. He was a casualty in the wasteland of unresolved soldier scars.

When he was almost fifty, the doctor came to unplug the machines that had been keeping him alive. The black cancer had spread to his lungs from his heart, leaving his entire chest cavity a shadow. He left behind lots of babies and a teenage wife who couldn't drive or read, and a reservoir of epigenetic pain.

Sometimes I see him in my dreams. He is dark and so am I. But my darkness is iridescent. I move lithely, but in a foreboding way as well. I am a large, sensual cat in the twilight. I am not here to hunt. I have come to protect and preserve myself, my cubs, the lineage that is now mine. I've come to retrieve something sacred and pure from a black hole of ancestral pain.

When our eyes meet, we hold the gaze until his black shadow shrinks from a scary man to a small boy. He is grandfather, and he is father. And he is the unloved son. I see it all spilling through time. His big, broken spirit pulses specks of red blood from a heart that used to beat. He is inside my ceremony because we share blood and epigenetics. He seeks salvation. He's done with the fight. Salvation is not mine to give, but there is something archetypal I can offer. As a mother now—embodied and unafraid—I tell him: "You're held accountable, but still forgiven. The struggle is done."

This man raised my father, the third of eight children who were born into poverty and chaos. Because there were so many of them and because their epic feuds ricocheted through the corn fields, nothing was secret in the way they wanted it to be. The shotgun rang out like a sheet of music to accompany the family score. They were violent, mad, and slightly wild— dark magic braided with raw potential. Add nurture, and anything could have changed.

My father made his way out of this wreckage by identifying two goals— stay sober and make money. His money created a different life for me, that's true. But his sobriety did not quell his rage. He lived from the haunted place that devoured love and left another kind of scarcity in its wake.

My dad's goals were well set before he met my mother. My mother was equally smart, but in different ways. She was an intellectual, not a survivalist. No trauma swirled inside her. By contrast, her idyllic childhood had left her with no sense of all that could possibly go wrong.

They bore me, not from violence, but neither with conscious intent. Love can also lead to accidental objects. This was my predicament. I was nestled between a mother who wanted a baby and a father who was terrified of passing on his pain. His rejection of me was a matter of his love, an attempt to protect me from himself. Their unconsciousness was almost my inheritance.

The child me needed someone to rescue and someone to blame. The adult me understands what the child could not. The trauma of growing up inside their tangles cultivated my intuition, and my ability to read people and the room.

I'm not the same kind of midwife my aunties were. But I've learned how to birth and rebirth certain things. How to take hurt and transmute it into something different. How to take the bitter and make it sweet. How to find the intersection at which shame and blame give way to empathy and forgiveness.

My canary song was both a lullaby and a scream. The answer to the riddle is to let love loom larger than fear. Replace caution with courage. The tiniest voice buried inside me was not so tiny after all. A tickle way in the back of my throat, followed by something that felt like choking. Ancestral hands constricting the airways, begging not to be silenced anymore. Then something that was half cough, half growl, barreled forward from the depths and what came out was my life. A story about moving from pious to righteous. A story being rewritten in real time.

Now, tell me, what will your story be?

YOUR TURN

What secrets do you keep? Who are you protecting? What is your true story? What are you waiting for to tell it? How would things be different if you could live in the truth?

JOURNAL PROMPTS AND REFLECTIONS

» Are you able to discern your ego's voice from your intuition? If yes, how do you tell the difference? What does intuition say or do differently than ego and vice versa?

» If you can't discern the two, what do you think is keeping you from that? Are you able to recognize multiple voices inside, or does it feel as if you're on autopilot, pulled in myriad directions without knowing why?

» Are there times when you think that it's better for ego to be in charge?

» What would a healthy new normal relationship between ego and intuition look like?

» How does understanding the function of those two internal voices inform life?

PART III

Integration

You do not have to be good.
You do not have to walk on your knees
For a hundred miles through the desert repenting.
You only have to let the soft animal of your body
Love what it loves.

— Mary Oliver

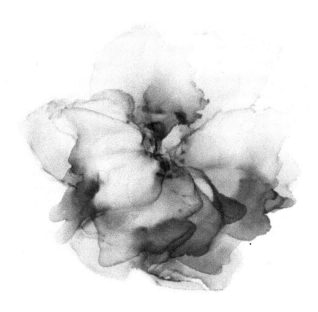

20

Birth Out of Crisis

*And the day came when the risk to
remain tight in a bud was more painful
than the risk it took to blossom.*

— Anais Nin

AS WE MOVE INTO PART III, our exploration shifts to the culminating stage of the psychedelic healing journey—*integration*. In these remaining chapters, my intent is to reveal the brutal truth of what it looks and feels like to live in the bumpy, beautiful aftermath of unearthing trauma and rebuilding your sense of self. Integration is often the hardest part of the journey. Yet somehow, it's discussed and understood the least. People fear the "bad trip" when, in fact, it is landing back in reality that is typically far more uncomfortable than the ceremony itself. But this is precisely what makes integration the biggest opportunity for growth. It is where the new awareness derived from the psychedelic space translates into lasting change—when we're willing and supported in doing the work.

As we've already seen, it is wise to orient ourselves to what's ahead. We must also understand that there is no way to know exactly what we'll need until we've arrived. A core part of integration is about beginning to exist in the present. In the late 1960s, psychologist Richard Alpert—now known as the beloved spiritual guru Ram Dass—traveled to India. His travels, his studies, and his psychedelic experiences emerged in a book called *Be Here Now* that was pivotal to the first psychedelic renaissance and reverberates now with even greater resonance.[7] Integration is precisely this endeavor—letting go of ruminations about the past and fixations on a future that is beyond our control, so that we may arrive in the present and *be here now*.

When we land in integration, we realize that the psychedelic medicine is not an end point or cure, but the beginning of a much longer journey that lies ahead. This central theme weaves like a vine throughout this book. To be in right relationship with powerful psychedelic medicines requires that we understand that they are not here to be used as a bypass around pain. Rather they bring us deeper into the core of what hurts. They are potent catalysts that require us to look deeply at even the hardest truths. Integration is about consciously choosing to write new stories in the face of these hard truths. To chase the ceremony is irreverent. Rather, we must bring the ceremony back to our lives. This requires a deepened awareness of how much work waits on the other side of the psychedelic session.

Most people emerge from ceremony feeling half-way reconstructed and highly disoriented. This is the felt sense of neurogenesis—dizzying possibility, heavy awareness, and a strong sense of responsibility. While neurogenesis and new stories is what we wanted, it rarely unfolds as we expected. We almost always feel worse before we feel better.

In the chapters that follow, you will gain glimpses into what is required to translate the sacred, ephemeral aspects of the psychedelic space into your reality. Several key themes emerge as anchors to stability throughout this tenuous period, but first, we must understand that coming out of ceremony is not as romantic or transcendent as it's been depicted.

I've yet to encounter a person on this path who transitioned out of the psychedelic space without one or all these experiences: a sense of existential crisis, a dark night of the soul, a need to withdraw and form new boundaries, a profound awareness of grief, as well as myriad other emotions that had been squelched along the way. When we've spent decades disassociating and/or controlling, the initial resurrection of strongly felt somatic experiences and emotions can be wonderful and totally overwhelming at the same time. We may have moments when we question everything—including the psychedelic path itself.

This makes conscious consent critical. Even at the hardest moments of integration, when we have said "yes" to the journey, it helps us shift away from victimization and lean deeper into agency. We can't "unknow" something once we've seen it through the psychedelic lens. We can't put the genie back in the bottle once it's out. When a spirit begins to free itself from conditioning, dogmas, and the pain of the past, it's not going to want to return to the smallness and pain of how things were before. But while not returning is certain, the path forward is not.

The landscape of integration is a long journey home to the wisdom of the wild and free within ourselves and the natural world. With time and support, integration provides an opportunity to bring love and honor to even the deepest wounds. Gradually, we stop trying to maneuver around our pain and begin to lean into the discomfort of facing what is there. As the great poet Rumi says: "The only cure for the pain is the pain." As much as we have tried to escape what hurts, integration is about facing and loving our hurt until it begins to transform before our eyes. In navigating this beautiful, difficult terrain, we restore innocence and hope to the child within ourselves and begin to live from a place of trust more than fear.

Crisis

My metamorphosis began in a hospital, under glaring lights, without my full-bodied consent.

The surgeon marched into my hospital room, smug and chipper. I disliked him already. He'd been analyzing my case with other doctors in front of me for six weeks. Six weeks of treating me like a science project rather than a human being. Forty plus days of addressing me as if I were a problem to solve, not a person in his care.

"You're going to meet your baby today," he said with the arrogance of a demigod, smiling with condescension. "Now, don't look so scared. This is a good thing."

I disliked him even more as he said this. How little this man knew of me. He'd never even bothered to ask. By this particular day, before he sliced me open, I'd already met my child many times on the astral plane. But this was not a language the demigod would understand.

I wanted to scream and throw things. How dare this man in his white coat—this man who had never birthed a baby himself—dare to speak with such hubris and flippancy? This same man had pummeled me with worst-case scenarios and insisted on every medical intervention to control my body and my baby for weeks on end. Now he demanded even my optimism—the same optimism he'd repeatedly doused.

Seconds after his declaration, they injected medication through an IV. No one asked permission. They shoved a consent form in my hands and urged me to sign with palpable desperation. No one acknowledged the obvious departure from ensuring that I was *actually okay* with what was happening, although some of the nurses mumbled something apologetic through pursed lips. Consent is so much more than a signature demanded under stress, or a muffled "okay" under squelched breath. But I was in no position to push back. I wasn't even fully lucid or in my body. I was a scared animal under attack.

Our birth playlist hummed in background, tethering me to the 233 days prior in which I had sung to this little spirit growing inside me. Our journey wasn't as I imagined, but it was no less a portal to possibility. In the operating room, a sterile triage procedure unfolded at the hands of scared and scary men hunting for control and self-preservation. They operated, perhaps with good intentions, in a space that transcended their intellectual comprehension. Puffed up with self-importance from their world of technical, scientific training, they lacked reverence for Mother Nature's design.

After multiple weeks in the hospital and then three more in the neonatal intensive care unit, those same doctors sent us home. The professionals said we were great. We had a clean bill of health—me and my tiny three-pound preemie, although I was in the midst of a post-partum crisis. They declared our greatness with the same arrogance and misguidedness they had used when they had insisted on our consent to slice me open. Never mind everything that had just happened. Never mind that my baby wasn't strong enough to breast feed. Never mind that my body was producing milk for two, including the "vanishing twin" who didn't make it. Never mind the PTSD flashbacks that were starting to emerge. Never mind the crushing fear that my mind was falling apart. No one even asked about my mental health.

Instead, they sent me out of the hospital barely stitched together with prescriptions for pain and post-partum mania. They praised themselves for saving us with all their modern interventions. They weren't all wrong, but they certainly weren't all right. What they missed was perhaps what mattered most—my mental health, my sense of agency, my baby's need for a supported mother.

When I returned home, I didn't feel like the same person who'd left. I'd been through hyperemesis, two placental abruptions, and preeclampsia. While statistically rare, my case of preeclampsia didn't resolve post-delivery, but required further medical intervention. By the time my son was in my arms a day and a half after delivery, I'd been told consistently to prepare for all kinds of risks—including, worst of all, that he could die. If there's anything to make a mother lose her mind, it's the thought of losing her child. I was compromised, to say the least.

My husband was supportive, but shell-shocked. After nearly two months of signing waivers and making massive decisions with urgency, we were both respectively ungrounded. I had an emerging resentment toward him that I didn't yet understand. I felt disconnected and estranged. He had gone home at nights, while I stayed in the hospital. Although I was the one who encouraged him to go, some part of me felt abandoned every time he left. Without him there, it was just me and my baby in that most alarming place on earth watching the clock tick. I didn't even have the presence of mind to recognize how terrified I was. I was too busy being brave.

There was something about the intense fragility of my post-partum body and everything we'd gone through that forced an opening into all that was unresolved in my past. At home, I was paralyzed by fear. My body was in physical shock and pain. I had multiple bouts of mastitis from the massive quantities of milk my body produced for a child barely big enough to nurse. I was fatigued beyond belief, but determined not to close my eyes. We didn't have alarms at home like they had in the hospital. What if I shut my eyes for a second and his little body forgot to breathe? How would I know if something happened unless I stayed awake? I managed to make it seven days straight without sleep. With each day, I became increasingly manic and paranoid. When sheer exhaustion finally took over, I woke to violent nightmares. Flashbacks from abusive scenes of childhood that had been successfully buried until now emerged at what felt like the least convenient moment.

I'd been conditioned for as I long as I could remember to fear my body. Now it seemed as if it was living up to the patriarchal promise. The evangelical story of Eden shoved down my throat as a child had forecast this pain and bloodshed, along with a promise of punishment for being female. The reckoning, I was taught, was menstruation and childbirth. The message was: *This is going to hurt.* My experience had been especially bloody and painful, which made me feel as if I was especially bad. We'll talk more in the next chapter about the connection between psychology and physiology, but what happened in my pregnancy mirrored what I felt and believed deep down about my body. It was fundamentally flawed, and I was going to suffer.

YOUR TURN

What is your relationship to crisis? What resources do you have for support? What is your understanding and/or perception around how psychedelics work and how long this journey will take?

Metamorphosis

Several months later, hanging on by a thin thread, I stepped into one of my first psychedelic sessions. Within minutes of the medicine taking effect, the scene of my son's birth and all the related beliefs about punishment were exactly what the medicine revealed. I saw myself trembling in that freezing operating room, so exposed and vulnerable under the fluorescent lights.

Big men in blue paper gowns with sharp sterile objects hovered around me speaking in a language I couldn't understand.

In the psychedelic space, however, I heard a different voice in that room—a strong and maternal voice, a calm and soothing voice. "You are never not in my hands, especially here. My design is a prism of possibilities. Each soul chooses its destiny. Now, go," the Earth Mother said. "Rebuild this memory"

A thousand pixels began to shift and rearrange as I heard these words. Slowly, a new picture replaced the old one that was frozen in the belief that my body had failed and that I was deserving of punishment. I entered that place a maiden and exited a mother.

They say a portal opens when a spirit comes through and, for a moment, we can reach into the next dimension. I felt that energy when I saw my baby pulled from my stomach, blue and barely strong enough to cry. This was the ending of life as I'd known it and the beginning of a new one. What looked like crisis was a necessary death. Something inside me knew, even in that most vulnerable moment, that my child and I were not going to persist in an intergenerational story of being broken. Not on my watch. We were born to heal and feel, however hard that might be. It was not too late for me to learn, or too early for my child to arrive. We were just in time. And the catastrophic experience we had just been through was somehow part of the karmic design.

That great maternal voice instructed me to listen and learn, and, above all else, to trust that I was not alone. In shattering silence, I heard a voice that came both from inside and outside myself.

"Look all around, child," the Earth Mother said. "The answers are waiting in my world. Everywhere you turn, you will find me. You want to know how to play with your baby. Look at my otter splashing with her pups in the water. Can you hear their laughter? Can you feel their joy?

"Are you afraid to show your fierceness because it might hurt your child? Watch my lioness with her cub when it steps beyond the den. This is an education in love and boundaries, perfect and complete. Watch closely as she takes him by the scruff. See her firm shake before nuzzling him back to her beautiful body. The lioness doesn't hesitate in owning her power. Her power is his safety.

"Go, walk wild, fierce, and happy into your life."

Deconstruction and Rebirth

My first pregnancy and birth experience marked the beginning of deconstructing everything that had been "patriarchalized" inside myself. It marked the end of my maiden voyage and the beginning of discovering what it meant to be an embodied mother. All the systems and adversaries I had been too scared to face before I became a mother, I was unwilling to ignore for my son. What I thought led me down the psychedelic path and what I discovered were both intimately connected, and miles apart.

Considering what we know now about epigenetics and intergenerational trauma, there are really no surprises in my story. Even the most awful things could have been predicted. Understanding this was more hopeful than sad, because it meant I had the capacity to change what was broken in my lineage by starting with myself. This is exactly what psychedelic neurogenesis and transferential support have made possible. The capacity to change my mind, as it turns out, was not a myth. Pretending to you or anyone that it's been easy—that would be unethical and a lie. Challenging as it was, however, I would do it all over again.

My son's birth catalyzed my psychedelic rebirth. I emerged from the hospital in an existential crisis. I felt more alive and myself than ever before, but, at the same time, as if part of me were dying. None of the coping mechanisms I'd cultivated over twenty years of trying to control my life with hypervigilance were going to work anymore. Counting calories and restricting my diet while producing massive amounts of breast milk wasn't even possible. Keeping the house in pristine order—not a chance. I couldn't go back, and I wasn't sure how to proceed. As uncomfortable as that felt, it was exactly where I needed to be. This is how integration begins, as a crisis of coming into consciousness after a deep sleep.

My daily intention was to find the magical mess of my deconstructed identity and illusions. My daily mantra was: *I'm powerfully in my process.*

These two anchors, supplemented with a village of care, slowly but steadily started to rearrange my reality. Many days in the beginning looked like disaster, but deep inside the heart space, love was beginning to grow even alongside the residue of pain.

JOURNAL PROMPTS AND REFLECTIONS

» Imagine yourself in limbo. Things are not under your control. Describe everything about how that feels. Let yourself flow with stream of consciousness. Don't edit.

» Imagine your life one year from now. If things were better, if you felt better, how would life look different? How would it feel different? Describe that picture.

21

Where Body and Mind Meet

*When a child is born, the entire Universe
has to shift and make room. Another entity
capable of free will, and therefore capable
of becoming God, has been born.*

— Ina May Gaskin

WHEN WE EMBARK ON A PSYCHEDELIC HEALING JOURNEY, our awareness of our body-brain connection awakens and reconstructs. The place where my physiology and my psyche collided was dramatically illuminated by the traumatic nature of the birth experience I described in the last chapter. Up to that point, my entire life had been mentally managed, while I remained wildly disassociated from my physical frame. Post-pregnancy and birth, my body screamed for attention and repair. I fumbled to find a new equilibrium.

Perhaps it was the messy aliveness I now felt in my body that gave me a sense of possibility. Perhaps it was the imprint of my ancestors, all of whom had had many babies. It's hard to say. But much sooner than expected, I started to long for another baby. Nothing about the desire was rooted in logic. My body and spirit said "yes," but my brain was terrified of what could go wrong. I was barely on solid ground after my last pregnancy. Now I had a little son to care for as well. What if all the complications happened again?

It didn't feel so much like having something to prove—more like a deep knowingness within. I'd met my first son in my dreams before he was born. Now, my youngest son started talking to me in my sleep. Whenever I tuned in to listen to that little baby spirit, I heard a strong, soft, and clear voice saying: "*It will be different this time.*"

All the doctors from what I call the "catastrophe ward" insisted that having another child was incredibly risky, even foolish. When I told them I wanted to have the child naturally, one of them laughed at me. "A vaginal birth after a Cesarean is utterly out of the question," she said, piercing a part of my feminine potential with her words. But despite what the white coats in their sterile hospital said, I knew that there was more than adequate evidence of women giving birth naturally after having had a C-section.

To add insult to injury, the white coats also told me to wait at least two to three years to ensure that my body was strong enough to try again. Then they said that the complications I had experienced were a result of my being too old—at the ancient age of thirty-six. None of the experts could agree on anything—except that natural birth was entirely out of the question for me. They were all appalled when I said that I'd decided to work with a midwife instead. The audacity! To give myself this chance in the face of all their experience and expertise!

Learning to Trust

I reached out to the midwife who was supposed to have delivered our first baby before the complications began, hoping that I hadn't spoken too soon. She had remained in touch with me even when I was no longer technically her patient. She sent me a bouquet of flowers after my C-section to welcome my baby into the world and congratulate me on becoming a mother. Her's was the perspective I wanted most, because I trusted her in a way I couldn't even begin to develop with the other doctors. She was a naturopathic physician as well as a midwife. Although I wasn't certain, I suspected that she might have a different take on how to proceed.

I will never forget her response to my questions: "Micah, I trust your body." Her simple words reverberated to my core. She could have stopped there, and it would have been enough. But as she continued, I felt goosebumps rise on my skin. "The female body is an incredible thing. Birth doesn't have to go badly every time. We can be careful and monitor things, and the hospital is right next door if you need it."

No one had ever trusted my body before. My body had been a problem from the moment I had been born a girl and not a boy. It was sterilized and objectified throughout adolescence. I was taught that my emerging sexuality was a vile thing that needed to be controlled. It was broken with infertility and a series of emergencies throughout a pregnancy that the medical world called a disaster. The pervasive message was that, in the absence of control, bad things—dangerous things—would happen. The notion that my body could be trusted was revolutionary to me.

I wanted to experience a natural childbirth. I had ravenously consumed every Ina May Gaskin book available during my first pregnancy and was unraveling the thread of midwifery in my lineage. Gaskin, who was known as the Mother of Midwifery, had started the sustainable commune in Tennessee called Summertown with her husband.

Summertown was a legendary place in my childhood terrain, a unique pocket in the otherwise repressive South from which artists and freethinkers emerged. Gaskin suggested that the whole model of birth in a hospital was designed for the doctors' convenience far more than a mother's ease. The energy of birthing she described felt known somewhere deep in my body. I wanted the sacredness of that experience myself. I wanted to reclaim a thing I didn't fully comprehend—the immeasurable power of the feminine body. I had had enough of the catastrophized or commodified dogma put forward by the patriarchy.

My partner and I gave it a lot of thought, and decided to trust. If complications emerged, we knew what to do. We'd been down that road already. But what if it went differently this time? How amazing would that feel?

How healing would that be? Given how long it had taken to get pregnant the first time (I'd needed fertility drugs), we decided not to wait.

Much to our surprise, I got pregnant on the first attempt with no interventions needed. We got the good news on Father's Day. My son was born nine months later on my husband's fortieth birthday as snow fell softly outside the window of the birth center.

Getting pregnant naturally, without intervention, felt like evidence that my DNA was re-assembling—as if my body wasn't broken after all. I had no placental abruptions or preeclampsia. I passed each milestone with a sense of relief and empowerment. Giving birth according to nature's design was the most wildly wonderful psychedelic experience of my life, a profound instruction on trust and surrender.

Despite being cautioned against it, my second child was born entirely naturally in the most painful and transformative ways. If I'd listened to the "experts" instead of my intuition, I'd have had a second C-section just to be safe. In so doing, I would have moved farther away from my intuition and potentially deepened the disassociation in my body. I'm not discounting the merits and necessity of interventions at times. But I am challenging the speed with which we default to "cut and control." I am inviting a more critical consideration of holistic care. I'm advising women to actually trust, rather than control, their bodies.

YOUR TURN

How do you resource yourself? How has your understanding of self-care evolved as you've read this book and navigated your healing so far? What techniques do you regularly use to self-soothe?

Holistic Care

We do something very similar in mental health. Traditional medical models advocate a quick recourse to prescribed medications to manage symptoms without getting to their root cause. In so doing, they add layers of complexity and create a dependency on medications that might not even address the core issue. Rather, they compound problems by adding serious side-effects. Even in psychedelic work, the medicines work by taking us deeper to the root of trauma, which facilitates healing. But if our bodies have been physiologically altered due to chronic stress and anxiety, it will take more than psychedelics to stabilize blood pressure or balance the thyroid. That's why it's critical that, in the mental-health context, we take a holistic approach if we're going to help people heal.

New possibilities are housed in the overlapping space where the body and mind meet. The physiological shift I experienced from my first pregnancy to my second is directly related to working through the core of my trauma. Epigenetics is helping us understand this profound connection between our physiology and our psychology—between nature and nurture. To be explicit, I'm not saying that psychedelic therapy healed my fertility issues or made it possible for me to have a natural childbirth. I don't have statistical research to make that case. I'm just one person. But if you asked me if I thought deep psychedelic and transferential work impacted my body as much as my psyche, the answer is absolutely and resoundingly "yes."

Autoimmune dysfunction and disease don't just suddenly appear, even if the diagnosis lands as a surprise. When we trace through patients' histories, we often find a through line of trauma begging for support. In the absence of that support, a body that's been relentlessly striving will eventually run out of stamina. It will come to a point when it can't persist. This is when we start to see physical symptoms emerge. It is also the moment when we feel most upset, or even betrayed by our bodies, as I initially did during my first pregnancy.

The only true solution to this is holistic care. Rather than trying to diagnose and control, holistic health systems and practitioners view symptoms as invitations to explore root causes and provide holistic treatment. This is how my naturopathic midwife approached my pregnancy. She didn't assume or default to a worst-case scenario before it even happened. She gave my body a chance, and gave me supplemental support. She brought a comprehensive understanding of my overall health history to my entire pregnancy. The combination of emotional and physiological support had a huge impact on my sense of safety and, in turn, my capacity to relax and trust my body.

Laboring to deliver a child is a perfect metaphor for the healing journey. It is excruciating and almost unbearable. But it is absolutely, utterly worth it. As a result of two entirely different experiences of bringing life into the world, the numbness that had dominated my body and my life was shattered. For thirty-eight years, my body had been labeled as the problem. Giving birth naturally gave compelling evidence that my body was capable of just about anything. My second birth helped me understand what is possible with holistic support, even when we've faced our deepest darkness. True trauma repair happens at this intersectional space where physiology and psychology come together as one.

I see the exquisite beauty in each of my son's birth stories, and the reflection of my own rebirth and healing through them. One was not "better" than the other. Rather each was a mirror in which I could see where I was in my own healing. Each was a catalyst to help me deepen and grow. Our children are our greatest teachers. Each of my birth journeys made silencing the primordial scream inside myself not only unnecessary, but impossible, although in different ways. As I birthed my babies from my womb into the world, my voice shifted from an apologetic whisper to a roar.

JOURNAL PROMPTS AND REFLECTIONS

» Consider the things you've already tried in your healing path. Make a list. What worked? What didn't?

» Now try to tune in to your intuition to learn how you resource yourself? How has your understanding of self-care evolved as you've pursued your healing journey? Have you developed more ways to self-soothe?

» Try to capture more nuance of what made a certain practice work or not work. Was it the practitioner? The modality? The space?

» Consider the places/spaces in nature that feel most nurturing to you. Describe a scene or experience there and then
   take yourself to that space every morning and/or evening.
   Sometimes finding a blueprint for safety inside yourself happens better in the natural world than in a clinical setting.

» Write about a time when you felt most embodied. Include
   all the sensory details you can recall.

22

Beyond the Binary

*You see, when the world becomes too solid for
nuance, when it hardens up and crystallizes
into a binary that forces you to pick a side,
compelling you to become intelligible to
the hardness that creeps on its once loamy
surfaces, cracks become the first responders.*

— Báyò Akómoláfé

THE ENDEAVOR TO HEAL FROM PTSD AND CPTSD is wrapped up in our capacity to step out of binary thinking into more expansive possibilities. This is challenging, because one of the most common byproducts of trauma is movement away from the natural childlike state of curiosity and wonder to one of being constantly on alert. Over time, this preoccupation with safety expresses itself in several different ways. It can become an almost manic mental management of details and anticipation. This might present as obsessive-compulsive behaviors or as an extreme fixation on control. Some people become highly disassociated—"checked out" of their lives— while others alternate between the two poles of vigilance and disassociation. Hanging in the balance is a mind stuck in the rigid binary mode of either/or thinking. Change is hard to experience from that reductionistic perspective.

This is one of many reasons why psychedelic medicines in the right set and setting can have such a profound impact. The neurogenesis they catalyze creates movement in the rigidity of thoughts. New synapses are formed. New possibilities emerge. Rigidity gives way to openness. With time, curiosity returns. As I described in earlier chapters, we can watch this neurological activity on brain scans taken of people under the influence of psychedelics. I've also witnessed it in sessions with my clients. The somatic clues are visible. Breathing patterns become steadier. Posture and facial expressions soften. Sometimes people tremble or twitch. Each of these somatic expressions reflects the body's movement out of a chronic state of fight-or-flight.

It is very hard, if not impossible, to replicate something we haven't felt. For many of my clients, the capacity to relax, to stop working and simply trust, is a completely foreign concept when they begin the psychedelic journey. But held in a village of care, with the right medicines, the nervous system has a chance to remember what it feels like to step out of the fight-or-flight binary state and land safely back home in life.

Jack's Homecoming

Jack was visibly distressed within minutes in our first online session. Through watery eyes, he told me: "I don't want to die with all this pain. I want to take something else to the other side." At that moment, he was struggling to get out of a wheelchair.

Jack was a sixty-eight-year-old filmmaker who was suffering from a condition called *ataxia*, which presented as a sudden loss of muscle control. The doctors ran a battery of tests, but couldn't find anything to explain the symptoms, which seemed to have come out of nowhere. They attributed Jack's condition to old age and prescribed a cocktail of medicines that caused an onslaught of side-effects—for each of which, of course, they prescribed a new medication. But Jack still felt terrible physically and even worse psychologically.

As he began to share his story, I was astounded by the depth and scope of trauma he'd endured throughout the journey of his life, and the incredible amount of resilience that must have been required just to stay alive. Jack had lived through harrowing childhood abuse and neglect. He left home at seventeen after being rejected for his sexuality in an era when being gay in the South was not acceptable. He survived the streets of New York City during the '60s and '70s, the peak of the first psychedelic renaissance. He watched countless friends die of AIDS.

He made repeated attempts to reconcile with a family who shunned and shamed him for who he was. Yet the little boy inside still longed for love, secure attachment, and a safe place to call home and be seen. As I listened to him recount his life experiences, I could hardly fathom the inner strength it must have taken to have endured so much abuse and pain. But here he was—still unwilling to give up on life's potential.

"Psychedelics are a homecoming to me," he told me. "I was there for the first psychedelic movement. I want to be part of this one. That was the only time in my life I recall feeling as if maybe all these unbearable experiences weren't totally my fault." Now the success of clinical trials was substantiating and validating his distant memories.

On the brink of a devastating break up and debilitating symptoms, Jack was ready and willing to try anything. Because his trauma was so complex and deep, because he couldn't remember much from his childhood, we intentionally went slowly in the preparation process. He told me repeatedly that part of him wanted to believe he could get better, but that most of him felt it was a lost cause. He flip-flopped between believing he'd get better and believing he'd die in the process of trying. He remained in this binary back-and-forth state for over a year.

In ceremony, Jack got glimpses of hope that maybe his life could be different, but they were hard to hold once he landed back in real time. Because he had been shamed and scapegoated so much throughout his life, the hardest thing of all was for him to see himself as worthy of love and peace. Ever since he was seventeen, he'd been surviving, not living. Now he wanted to live. But there was so much standing in the way of that.

One of many things that kept Jack in a survivalist state was that, when he began his journey, he knew intellectually that he had trauma, but his actual memories felt disconnected, foggy, not his own. Because he couldn't remember his past, he struggled to trust himself. Chronic gaslighting by family members desperately seeking to cover up their own guilt and deny responsibility only made matters worse. His brain was trapped in a binary dislocation of a haunting past and an elusive future.

Because of the many physical symptoms Jack was experiencing, it was essential for his safety that we build a village of care and ensure that he had holistic support before proceeding. While building that team wasn't easy, I was surprised at how organically it came together. Jack found a psychologist who was completely open to psychedelic therapy (even in the conservative South). He found an endocrinologist to assess autoimmune pathologies and issues related to his ataxia. He got a physical therapist and Qi Gong master to work on flexibility and strength. He was more committed than perhaps any client I'd ever seen. His commitment and hope outweighed his fear, even on the hardest days. Throughout the whole journey, he remained unwavering in his original intention to complete the journey of his life with something beyond excruciating pain.

In one of our preparation sessions, Jack shared his feelings about being in a wheelchair. It was one of the most astounding, insightful things a client had ever said to me: "I can't help thinking this whole disability is somehow a way to hide from my life—the life I so desperately want to live and am equally terrified to face. There's got to be another way. I'm willing to try anything."

While it was never an explicit goal that Jack's healing would be defined or realized by his getting out of the wheelchair, I wondered what might be possible with his physical body as his spirit and psyche started to heal. I'd heard stories among indigenous healers about miraculous physical shifts that occurred as metaphysical pain was alleviated. To say that Jack's healing path was transcendent and beautiful would be both accurate and grossly misrepresentative.

─────── YOUR TURN ───────

What either/or scenarios get stuck on repeat in your mind? In your life? Can you imagine a picture beyond the binary? What might that look like and how would it feel different? In what unconscious ways does reducing things to either/or thinking help you play "safe?"

Breaking Free

Before beginning his psychedelic healing journey, Jack couldn't emerge from fight-or-flight mode because he had no memory of anything else. He couldn't break free of his binary, reductionistic thinking any more easily than he could have stepped out of his wheelchair. Rather, his process was iterative and gradual.

When we started working together, Jack had a system he'd been using since childhood to calculate "good days" and "bad days." For any good day, there had to be a certain number of bad days to balance it out. He'd imposed so many arbitrary rules on himself just to give himself a sense of control. But now he was trapped inside those rules. The rigidity and structure his mind had had to cultivate to stay alive was incredible. He had a whole battery of brilliant adaptive strategies to help him survive. But now those very strategies made him feel trapped inside himself.

Throughout his journey, no matter how hard or painful, Jack persisted. I watched him as—step by step, session by session, month by month—he took back his life. He set boundaries with abusive relationships. He reclaimed memories and processed enormous grief. At a turning point a little over a year into our work together, we both agreed that perhaps the good was finally there to stay. Maybe he didn't have to count good days and bad days anymore. Maybe they could all be okay. Maybe he was finally safe.

Gradually, Jack moved from a wheelchair to a walker. Then to a cane. He brought his cane with him when he came to Mexico to see me, but he returned home walking without it. I want to be explicit about this. I'm not saying that Jack's work with psilocybin and ketamine cured his ataxia or made it possible for him to walk again. There's no way to prove that. And that's not really the point. The point is rather that it was what Jack had realized himself that had the greatest impact of all—that being in a wheelchair was a way to hide from life when the world felt too scary to face. When he broke free of the binary traps—when he processed decades of trauma and allowed himself to grieve—everything changed for him. His physics and his metaphysics.

There were plenty of setbacks along the way, including more ataxia episodes. Each one brought Jack back to a familiar state of fight-or-flight. And every time, the doctors found no medical cause. And every time, Jack got back up—not through force or will, but rather from love. Despite all the trauma and abuse, and the complexity that he had created around loving himself, Jack somehow maintained his capacity to see and love the beauty that is possible in life.

Jack and I continue to work together today, just over two years after our initial online session. We've worked virtually and in person, in altered states of consciousness and in everyday 3-D time. Today, Jack rides a bike. He has two dogs that he walks daily in the dog park. He has reclaimed a world of haunting, painful memories in which his sense of the possibilities of life had been literally trapped. He's a living embodiment of what neurogenesis can yield.

When I told Jack about this book and asked if he'd be comfortable with me sharing his story, he said tearfully: "If it can help one person feel less alone, to have some kernel of hope to hold on to, then by all means, let's share it." When I asked him the single most significant shift that had occurred in his consciousness as a result of having navigated this experience, he replied: "For sixty-eight years, I lived in a painful reductionistic binary world. Either I would live, or I would die. Either I would take this pain to the grave, or I'd find freedom. Either I'd walk again or be in a wheelchair forever. Now I live in a space of possibility and expansion. My life isn't pain-free or perfect, but the good is here to stay."

JOURNAL PROMPTS AND REFLECTIONS

» Spend time journaling on multiple paths for your life. Envision each path with as much sensory detail and nuance as possible. Notice how all the paths have good things and bad things about them.

» Write a letter to the little child version of yourself. How can you help that child understand the things the grown-up you struggles to hold and know? What can you say to help that child understand that mistakes are necessary in order to learn?

» Consider a "mistake" you've made in your life. As you reflect on that now, describe how that mistake also led you to invaluable lessons.

23

Unblending

Who in the world am I? Ah, that's the great puzzle.

— Alice in Wonderland

ONCE WE'VE OPENED THE DEPTHS of our internal world with psychedelic therapy, we fall into what feels like a perpetual state of rearranging. Videogames in which every grasp at structure gives way to a new configuration provide a good analogy for how this integration can feel. It is a little like learning to stay balanced while life reconstructs itself in real time. In the beginning, this sense of structural instability can be overwhelming.

Think back to the internal family systems model and its operative concepts of protective, managing, and exiled parts, as well as the inner healer. When we experience trauma, our inner psyche splinters into different parts. This splintering is not bad; in fact, it is necessary to survival. Each respective part plays a unique role in keeping us safe, helping us develop strategies, habits, or beliefs to govern and control the chaos around us. The exiled parts are those we bury deep in our subconscious because they were most severely wounded by a trauma too crushing to face at the time. While these parts and methods were required to keep us safe, they perpetuate a survivalist mindset even when we no longer need them. They keep us from being open and receptive to possibility.

As we emerge from the psychedelic state, our most important protective parts and exiles are visible in a way they weren't before. Without this illumination, it's almost impossible to know where to begin with our healing. Protection has become so blended with our identity that we can hardly imagine a different life. All of this can feel a little like standing in a landslide being crushed by the chaos around you. While uncomfortable, however, it's this rearranging of the internal landscape that leads people to discover or remember their inner healer—that part within us that, when given a chance and resources, wants to heal and possesses an innate wisdom for how to go about it. For most survivors of PTSD or CPTSD, the protective, managing parts become so strong and the pain of the exiles is so vast that this inner healer gets eclipsed in the background.

Tapping into the wisdom of the inner healer is one of the most transformative components of the psychedelic therapeutic process. It's essential to understand, however, that reclaiming this wisdom within requires cultivation over time. Initially, as we emerge from the medicine space connected to our intuition, we want to live *only* in this connected space of clarity and resolve. But as we return to life's inevitable triggers, our devoted, well-cultivated protective parts come rushing back to the surface.

While this can feel frustrating in the moment and be experienced as regression, it is important to understand that the goal is not to *annihilate* any of our parts. Rather, healing is about honoring how our parts kept us alive and giving them permission to put down their burdens so they can relax. They can be there to support us when challenges or triggers appear, but they no longer need to dominate or limit our experiences. And that is when our inner healers can become more consistent leaders in our lives.

Unburdening Samuel

When I met Samuel, he was in the process of weaning himself off several pharmaceutical medications prescribed to help him manage his anxiety and depression. He had a two-year-old daughter and more reason than ever to be present in his life. Yet he reported feeling something I hear all too often—an overarching sense of numbness, a struggle to feel emotionally or connect to the things that mattered most to him. He was a classic over-achiever who felt perfection was required to be good enough and loved.

Samuel had been working with a colleague of mine for a few years who presented the idea of psychedelic therapy as a possibility with new potential and hope. Desperate to feel better, he was immediately receptive to the idea and we set up a consultation to discuss next steps. As I listened to him process his childhood, I noted common characteristics shared by other CPTSD survivors—a tendency to minimize how bad it had been, a tendency to defend caregivers, a struggle to remember childhood in any detail, and an overall disconnect from the somatic body accompanied by a constant tendency to analyze.

After discussion, we agreed that psychedelic therapy could be a way to help him open his emotions and be more present in his life with the people he loved. We also talked at length about how important it was to prepare for the experience and that he would almost certainly feel worse before he felt better. We settled on a preparation process of at least six sessions before considering moving into the medicine space. Initially, Samuel was interested primarily in psilocybin, because it was the psychedelic he'd heard the most about and because it was a natural medicine with an indigenous history and tradition. But he was open to other options.

As we worked through his preparation sessions, it was increasingly clear that Samuel was blended and identified with his protective parts, whose limiting beliefs were so strong that he struggled to access his inner healer. His layers of protection were so established that it was hard for him even to fathom a self-essence that wasn't on guard. The process of weaning himself off antidepressants was proving harder than anticipated, as is often the case. Add to this the real demands of parenting a fully embodied toddler, and he was feeling discouraged before we'd even gotten to the psychedelic part of the process.

Given this, I suggested that Samuel start with a series of low-dose ketamine sessions. Ketamine at low dose can be a gentle introduction to psychedelic therapy. It is also safe to use in conjunction with antidepressants, which is great news for many individuals struggling with depression. We agreed to do three sessions with the intention of getting to know and understand the parts in his internal family system better. We also set the intention to deepen the sense of safety and connection he felt with me as the person holding such a vulnerable space for him.

Samuel had a significant amount of attachment trauma related to his mother, which meant the opportunity for repair in the transferential space would be strong, particularly if we'd done a good job establishing trust in our dynamic. Knowing that he was incredibly analytical and spent an extensive amount of time lost in his thoughts, I knew that starting with a medicine like ketamine at a low dose would be less disorienting than a heroic dose of psilocybin. So we stepped into the psychedelic space with the intention of meeting and unburdening his internal family system.

YOUR TURN

Revisit the inventory of parts you identified in part I. How has your awareness or understanding of those parts already evolved? What new parts have you identified? In what ways were you confusing a part or parts with your inner healer?

Finding Balance

Five minutes into his first ketamine session, Samuel told me he thought he could feel his inner healer for the first time ever. "It's not that anything from my past is different from how I remember, but it all feels clearer and rearranged. What I thought I needed to heal and what is really the issue are not at all the same," he said, sounding surprised, but certain.

The story Samuel had been told since he was around five was that his father had abandoned him, his mother, and his brother for a life of drugs and alcohol. He thought his deepest healing revolved around that abandonment wound. But as he dropped deeper into his inner-healer wisdom, past all the protection, what was most striking was the way he'd spent his life emotionally supporting his mother. "I guess I have a mom wound, too.

This whole time I've thought it was all about my father," he said, seeming almost shocked at the discovery.

Over the next two ketamine sessions, we worked on deepening our transferential dynamic, which, as we saw in chapter 13, is one of the most potent variables in the psychedelic process because it allows a person to externalize memories, feelings, and experiences from childhood, making the relational space and container a canvas on which corrective experiences can be drawn. For Samuel, this unfolded in a series of subtle, but significant, reframings that created an opening in which he could begin to reconsolidate his sense of self.

When I asked him to imagine what it would feel like if his mother told him he didn't have to do anything to make her happy, a smile spread across Samuel's face and he replied: "I can't even imagine, but it sounds amazing." Then I suggested we try a little experiment. I repeated that thought: "All you have to do is be yourself. That is more than enough. You don't have to take care of your mom. She can take care of herself." I watched his body move in small twitches as he absorbed the possibility of not feeling so utterly responsible.

As we continued to work on unburdening some of Samuel's parts, a better understanding of his internal world emerged. With the supportive shifts made possible through this work with ketamine, he was able to successfully wean himself off his antidepressant medication. Despite the challenges of resurrecting the past, he was feeling for the first time ever, and his struggles and issues somehow made more sense.

By the time Samuel stepped deeper into the psychedelic journey with psilocybin, he had a much clearer picture of the parts in his internal family system. That clarity enabled further healing in the medicine space. In his first psilocybin session, he met the seven-year-old version of himself who had decided, given his mother's emotional fragility, that it was time to become the man of the house.

Because of the blurry nature of memories distorted by trauma, Samuel remembered some things about this experience in explicit detail and other things through a hazy fog. He recalled the specific car ride when he made that decision and how everything in his life pivoted after that moment. He remembered the song playing on the radio and the T-shirt he was wearing at the time. But he remembered nothing about his mother, apart from the overarching sense that he had to take care of her.

What was most surprising and amazing, however, was the flood of memories and details about his father that came back into focus as he acknowledged the pain and sacrifice connected to his mother. Suddenly, it was as if a hidden space opened in which he recalled going to the park with his dad and his dad pushing him on the swing. "I can feel his love," he marveled, totally surprised it was there. Nothing about this felt sense of his memory had been accessible to him before—not because the memory wasn't there, but because he was made to feel that acknowledging his father's love would be a kind of betrayal of his mother.

He also met the adolescent, young-adult version of himself who'd gotten tangled in a more complex web of enmeshment, one that reflected a different kind of caretaking. This part not only needed to take care of his mother in a generalized sense, but also needed to reassure her emotionally so she felt good about herself.

As his protective parts unburdened themselves and the memories came into focus, Samuel felt somatically the cost of being parentified. Remember that parentification is a painfully misunderstood expression of trauma in which the child takes on adult responsibility in numerous ways (see chapter 12). For Samuel, this almost overnight arrival at adulthood had caused panic attacks and debilitating migraines. Beyond physical symptoms, his enmeshment in his mother's emotional world cost him the innocence and play of childhood. His capacity to be curious, to rest, to explore—all these innate qualities of children disappeared, overridden by a need to be a responsible caretaker and partner. Wrapped up in all this was an understandable reservoir of anger that had been repressed, desperately needing to be released.

Deep in the mythopoetic psilocybin space, Samuel described a scene reminiscent of *Where the Wild Things Are*—a parallel, wild universe where he could be free and totally on his own. There was initial relief in finding himself in this other world, until he realized that, even here, far away, the Earth undulated. When I asked him what caused his world to shake, he answered without hesitation: "It's her. The sense of responsibility to take care of her needs makes my world unstable and shaky."

Out of the medicine space, Samuel's inner healer struggled to hold on to the balance of all his parts. In his unstable world, he toggled between a landslide of responsibility and a sense of self-preservation. In that space, his needs slipped through the cracks. Healing required that he put himself first, which he'd been conditioned to see as selfish and weak.

The endeavor to acknowledge felt needs and honor the parts within became the largest part of Samuel's integration work. He had to learn how to hold himself in balance in a shaky world and resist what had become an almost ingrained burden of responsibility. Integration was a gradual, ongoing process of learning how to disentangle his parts from his inner healer, and then establish a balance between them.

Samuel had to work with great intention and practice to release the pervasive sense of guilt his parts felt whenever he chose himself. It was not surprising that one of the most therapeutic integrative practices he discovered was going deep into the mountains to a rustic cabin with no Wi-Fi and no human contact—just the quiet solitude of himself. He had to unplug that much to rediscover himself.

With time, practice, and a village of care and support, Samuel was able to bring his unstable internal world into balance. From this place of balance, he also came to understand that each of his parts had played an integral role in his survival. He understood that the goal of his healing was not to make any of those parts go away, but rather to recognize them when they showed up.

Like many of us on the road to recovery from complex trauma, Samuel was able, through consistent integration, to untangle the knots inside himself. He took space from his mother. He took space to go into the woods to find himself. He showed up with great discipline to the endeavor of hoping that with time, love, and support, his life would feel different. While things continued to feel unstable periodically, he also began to play with his daughter. He started to explore his creativity. Gradually, he came to see his parts from his inner healer's perspective. From this point of balance, the multiplicity of parts became, not a problem, but a prism of possibility.

JOURNAL PROMPTS AND REFLECTIONS

» Consider a recent conflict through the lens of your inner healer. In what way were you blended when the conflict occurred? How would things have unfolded differently had you not been blended?

» What parts most needed unburdening in order to let your inner healer lead more easily?

24

Righteous Rage

Righteous anger is a tool of justice, a scythe of
compassion, more than a reactive emotion.

— Desmond Tutu

RIGHTEOUS RAGE IS ANGER THAT IS ROOTED in a desire for
healing, not in a desire to retaliate or perpetuate harm. It is righteous
because it fuels necessary change. To heal ourselves and our culture and
to help our children, we must reclaim our capacity to be honest and gen-
erative in our expression of anger. I regularly tell clients that righteous
rage is *love,* but those words are often met with a look of bewilderment
and confusion.

Without fail, all clients at some point in the healing journey arrive
at the impasse of their own rage. This rage shouldn't come as a shock,
yet it almost always does. Nor is this rage without cause. Rather, it is a
byproduct, an accumulation of micro- and macro-aggressions that have
been stockpiled over the journey of life. The root of this rage is bound
up in the somatic memory of violation, abuse, neglect, trauma, and pain
stored in the nervous system. The complexity of this feeling of rage, and
often why it gets buried, is that we exist in a culture that has made toxic
positivity a badge of honor.

Toxic Positivity

Healing requires us to resolve our anger into empathy and understanding—to move away from shame and blame and soften into forgiveness. Yet, there is no intellectual "bypass" that allows us to arrive at an earnest expression of forgiveness without first having fully processed our feelings. When processed constructively, in the right set and setting and with support, we can experience our rage as a welcome portal to new growth that is often wildly liberating.

The moment anger presents in the healing journey, things start to escalate and rearrange. Without fail, when the rage comes, everyone, at least initially, wants to look away. Our immediate impulse is to override rage with an intellectually sound reason why there's no substantial cause for it to be there. Meanwhile, the child inside is screaming and wants to have a tantrum while the adult is frozen at this impasse between their anger and their possibility.

Have you ever tried to reason with a child throwing a tantrum? Children don't care about logical explanations. Adults with a deeply wounded inner child are the same. They care about the immediacy of their feelings. If you want to have any chance of moving forward, you must first meet them in the context of their emotional outburst. Meet them in the emotion and hold space for them to feel. Then they can move forward. We can do this as adults as well, as we heal the child within. The work with psychedelics helps us gain access to the inner world of the child in order to repair.

A critical part of reaching children (or wounded inner children) involves acknowledging the validity of their feelings. Feelings are not logical. And like anything we consume, once metabolized, they can be digested and turned into material from which we can draw. But when feelings are judged or deemed as bad, they slow down the system, causing constipation, sluggishness, inflammation—both literally and metaphorically. They get stuck, like clogged pipes. Having emotions is not the problem. But repressing them is. Children who don't grow up in conscious, healthy homes with a full range of emotions learn to fear anger because it poses a threat to safety. This places an internal barrier around these feelings that makes naming them and tolerating them extremely challenging.

In our culture, we have come to label anger as bad and destructive, even toxic. Angry women are referred to as bitches, overly sensitive, hormonal. Angry men are characterized as violent, threatening, dangerous. What painfully reductionist ways to see an emotion so essential to catalyzing change! Certainly anger can be expressed in negative ways, unconstructively. But most often, this destructive version is rooted in repression, in an attempt to bottle up our anger rather than process it.

Countless times, I have heard clients recount a terrible story from childhood or their partnership and, within seconds, say something like: "Oh, but they're doing the best they can. They're trying. No point holding on to it." While that may be true and well-intentioned, when we say something like this, it invalidates our inner child and shames it for its emotions. Then, unintentionally, we start a cycle of blaming ourselves and struggling to trust. Imagine saying to a child who's being abused: "Don't be so upset. They're trying their best." While we can't imagine saying that to someone else, we say it to ourselves countless times.

What festers in the weeds of this toxic positivity is resentment, stuckness, and disembodiment. Until people get honest about their anger, they simply can't move forward. It is an impossible impasse.

Anger begins to surface most intensely in the integration stage of psychedelic-assisted therapy. Following an illuminating experience in the medicine space, people struggle to return to the stark incongruencies in their lives. This begins a period of reckoning and realignment of relationships, patterns, and dynamics that have been accepted as normal. In the aftermath of new awareness, what was once normal often stands out as glaringly dysfunctional. This creates friction, and that friction fuels anger.

For example, my family and I moved to Mexico amid a high-profile trial of a public figure accused of harrassment and sexual assault. While many variables informed our move, the rage ignited in the aftermath of revisiting a similar traumatic experience was an undeniable factor for me. As I watched witnesses relate their experiences of being raped with excruciating vulnerability and strength, a sense of rage I'd never allowed myself to acknowledge hurled to the surface. I vomited. I screamed. I cried. My body's physiological response resurrected the trauma within myself. We shared a collective wound of violation and nonconsent. I'd spent twenty years blaming myself for the occurrence in my own life. Now I retreated from a cultural context that made complicity not only acceptable, but encouraged.

Righteous rage has a visceral, somatic quality. It is a primal response that can fuel reaction and positive changes in our lives. Our capacity to stay in relationship to our anger catalyzes neurogenesis and growth. If we look away from it because it is frowned upon, this healing isn't possible. The somatic experience of allowing rather than suppressing righteous rage mirrors the psychedelic process. It opens something new.

YOUR TURN

Consider when/if you've experienced feelings of anger. How comfortable/uncomfortable was that experience? Consider if there are difficult things in your life that you find yourself rationalizing or minimizing. Consider how you respond to other people's anger.

The Memory Box

In the medicine space, I hear a question posed to me through a voice that sounds ancient, maternal, and safe: "My child, can you forgive yourself for being angry and imperfect? That is really the point. Can you love yourself the way I love you? Can you remember we're made of the same essence?"

Next, that maternal presence directs my gaze toward a memory box, a treasure trove of possibilities and pain where my internal family of parts resides. I recognize this box from childhood, wooden and intricate in design. I open it and a little ballerina girl spins while a familiar song plays in the background.

The first memory I find is sixteen-year-old me in tight jeans and a crop top. She's frail and skittish. She avoids my glance, but I can feel she wants to be seen. She needs help. She's like a street girl, tough and tattered, but fragile. She clutches a bag over her heart and her stomach.

As I try to approach her, she hisses. She doesn't trust me—my street girl part, covered in bruises. She's been through an ordeal. I see tear streaks through her makeup. She moves like a wounded animal in defense mode. She's angry, but no one has given her permission to feel anything. She looks at me as a child looks at its mom—for approval.

I realize in this moment that *I am her mom*, and she is me. This is another re-parenting moment come to life inside an altered portal of space and time. I tune myself to the emerging maternal part of myself. I look in this street girl's eyes. Gradually, her defenses dissolve. She drops her bag, revealing a gaping hole. The hole is the hollow of her pelvic bowl.

She tries to talk, first in a quiver. Until now, no one has acknowledged her or seen her. Her words initially are indiscernible, like animal sounds. Finally, she manages to say: "I was not numb. I felt everything. Every violence on your watch. Each hand that touched us the wrong way. I felt it all, and it crushed me. How can I trust you?"

We sit together, these two parts of myself. The girl and the woman. The woman, mom part is the newest to know. She feels ancient and connected. She has intuitive wisdom of what to do and how to create safety and repair, which is precisely what she does.

"I'm sorry for all of it, that no one told you how sacred you are. I see you. I'm here now. I'm not going away," I tell her.

What follows feels like waking from a dream. Speckles of gold flicker and shimmer in the air. This is the picture of safety I'd been searching for my whole life—not perfection, but complete possibility. Numbness stems from repressed anger. Clawing out of the barbed wire of our pain stories is an arduous, but worthy, endeavor. Wholeness waits in wonder in a native land that knows love is our birthright.

Softening into Time

When I began this journey, I saw healing as an endgame—some sort of commodity packaged and sold with a definitive finish line. I expected a strong return on investment with quick turnaround. With time, I've come to understand that the return on investment for my soul's resuscitation is immeasurable and totally beyond any capitalist metaphors.

I've come to realize that healing required that I stop playing certain societal games that kept me dishonest and disconnected from my body and myself. Societal games are everywhere and can seem innocent enough, until suddenly they are not. Chasing popularity on social media, fighting time through beauty treatments, or the pervasive expectation of immediacy dominant in today's world—these are just a few of the insidious traps that our current culture aggressively pounds into our minds and homes.

By contrast, the great curanderas have always held the wisdom of softening into time and the elements. They invite and encourage a safe space to hold all the wild and full range of embodied emotions. They understand that the medicine is woven into the wheel of life, not a thing to place on top of it. The goal is not to live for the ceremony, but to bring that vibration of ceremony to life. To reclaim what was lost or repressed and find that the resonance of righteousness can be possible in every feeling we can fully embody.

JOURNAL PROMPTS AND REFLECTIONS

» What would help create a sense of safety when expressing a challenging emotion like anger? If you knew there was no danger, what would you want or need to say?

» Do you have memories or experiences that you know make you angry, but you can't *feel* anything? Do you feel numb? Journal about the numbness and/or the memory and see what comes up.

» Now try focusing on that memory while doing something physical. How do you notice or experience the emotion? Less as an intellectual thought and more as a physiological process?

(25)

Nature as Medicine, Earth as Mother

The land knows you, even when you are lost.

— Robin Wall Kimmerer

WE HAVE ALREADY SEEN HOW INDIGENOUS TRADITIONS honor an intimate connection to nature and a solid connection to community. In this cultural ethos, secure attachment begins with our connection to the Earth. Plant medicines provide a conduit for tuning in to the Earth Mother's wisdom and voice, and for establishing an intimate relationship with the vast maternal presence of Pachamama, who governs the rhythms and cycles of the natural world. This relationship is integral to abundance in life and to living in right relationship with the Earth. Rather than celebrating autonomy or fierce independence, indigenous communities derive strength from an experience of community that is punctuated by ritual and ceremony that anchor daily life in the sacred.

It is this sense of secure attachment that is shattered by trauma in today's world. In the psychedelic space, we often learn that our first attachment injury occurred when, driven by trauma and the pressures of modern life, we disconnect from this elemental force. Because of this, many people find that their healing lies in a reconnection to nature. My mentor once told me that, in over 3,000 pschedelic-assisted healing sessions with clients, nature had come up as a solution in nearly every single one. These next two stories are good examples of that.

Just Listening

A couple years ago in the midst of the pandemic, a client contacted me to explore the possibility of working with psilocybin. He was a young man in his early thirties whose situation was a little bit different from my usual cases in that he didn't seem to have a backdrop of complex trauma. Rather, he had an isolated event that had impacted everything else in his life. When he was relatively young, an unexpected complication from a severe infection had resulted in significant hearing loss. He wanted to know if psilocybin and the neurogenesis it sparked could make his hearing come back. To be honest, I had no idea if that was possible, which is exactly what I told him.

He asked me to describe the most amazing change I'd seen come out of the psychedelic space. It was a hard question to answer, because I've seen many incredible things, some almost impossible to believe. I narrowed it down to a couple of possibilities, but, given that his issue was physical in nature, Jack came to mind (see chapter 22). As I shared Jack's story, I watched the young man's eyes light up with possibility. Sensitive to the potential of giving him false hope, I reminded him that I had absolutely no data or anecdotal evidence of any case like his in which psilocybin had been the cure.

Despite the absence of empirical evidence, however, I told him that, regardless of the outcome, I suspected that the experience itself would give him a new or different perspective on his relationship to his hearing. He looked less impressed with that response. After a couple of days reflection, however, he sent me this text: "I guess I really don't have anything to lose. I'd rather take the risk of disappointment than not try at all."

A handful of preparation sessions later, he arrived at my office for ceremony. It was the quietest ceremony I'd ever attended. Deafening silence filled the minutes and hours that slowly ticked by. I checked in periodically, making sure that all was well in the stillness, and each time, he gave me the most peaceful, contented nod. His face and body looked calm on the couch across from me. Sometimes it almost looked as if he were smiling. He was somewhere deep in the mycelium folds. After about four hours, he sat up straight and said to me: "I heard the water in the stream loud and clear."

Apparently, he'd gone hiking a few days before the ceremony. He didn't wear his hearing aids because he was with a girl he liked and felt self-conscious about them. On the hike, the thing that had stood out most for him was a beautiful stream that led to a waterfall that he could barely hear. It was only right at the water's edge, where the pressure mounted most, that he could hear the faintest sound in the distance. His life had grown to feel like this over the years—a thing he could almost hear and feel. Almost, but not quite.

But in his ceremony, he heard the stream. He heard birds and his favorite songs. He heard everything in full, complete resonance. "The sound is inside myself," he said tearfully. "I just need to listen."

YOUR TURN

Consider your relationship to nature. What moments or experiences stand out the most? How have you leveraged nature as medicine in your life? Do you have any rituals connected with or connecting you to the Earth?

Getting to the Root

Julie was a mother of three. Her sister struggled with addiction, and she had a complicated relationship with her parents. While initially reticent to say it, she suspected her mom might be a narcissist. Part of her felt dramatic or disloyal when she described her family of origin.

It was clear that Julie struggled with trusting herself. From our first consultation, I had the sense that there was more to her than what she was allowing me, or even herself, to see. She seemed guarded and a little nervous. It felt as if there was a part in her internal family system that was accustomed to being misunderstood and rejected. She was understandably on alert for that possibility in our sessions as well.

It was also clear that Julie wanted to engage in this psychedelic journey. She had been on a healing path for several years before we met, working to address autoimmune issues. Numerous protocols and a certification in functional health had helped her gain tremendous insight into how to better support her physiology. But she was still struggling. She'd come to the conclusion that, underneath everything dysregulated with her physical body, there was a root cause of unresolved trauma. Whether it was a looming sense of hypervigilance or an almost constant upset stomach, her body and her nervous system made it very clear that something needed to shift. She knew somehow that, even though all her memories of childhood were foggy, there was something she'd not yet been able to unearth. This was where our focus was going to be—getting to the root.

It's poetic that getting to the root was the focus, because the symbol of roots and trees presented in her first ceremony and in nearly every ceremony that followed. As the medicine began to work through Julie's system, she felt a wave of anxiety swim to the surface. We went through a meditation to help her soften into her body and her breath. As she came out of the meditation, her eyes fixed on a tree outside the window and she said: "It's as if it's communicating with me."

"Nature speaks," I responded. "We're here to remember how to listen."

She closed her eyes, looking very peaceful. The anxiety had clearly passed. Then she said: "I feel as if I can let the need to resolve everything with my parents go. It feels as if the Earth is my mother." She smiled and we sat together in the calm presence, the distant sound of leaves rustling through the tree.

Some time passed and Julie looked up again to tell me that she could see herself running alongside a river she remembered from her childhood. "We're running through the fields beside it," she told me. "I'm having so much fun here, but something changed, and I can't tell what it is."

I asked Julie to walk me through as much as she could remember. She'd been playing in the fields with a couple of her friends, one of whom happened to be a little boy. He was chasing them and at first it seemed fun, but then it felt scary. From the moment it got scary, Julie couldn't remember anything else. Her memory went that far with details, but the felt sense of fear was enough for her to know that something wasn't safe.

I told her to trust herself and her body and that she wasn't alone. I would be right there with her. I reassured her that it was okay if she didn't remember all the details.

I watched tears flow down Julie's cheeks. She stayed quiet for a while and, when she opened her eyes again, she told me: "I don't know what happened in that field, but I know I stopped playing after that. I stopped going outside. I lost that connection to nature. It's true. Losing that connection made everything harder."

Knowing that play is such an important part of being a child, I asked her whether she could take back some of her trust in the Earth, and whether that would make it easier to play now.

She closed her eyes again and, before she said another word, I could feel the energy shift around us. It felt like a breeze after a storm, fresh and clean. I wondered if Julie could feel it too. Right at that moment, she looked up and said: "It feels as if my ancestors are here. They're standing around a big tree and telling me I can give this pain back to the Earth. The Earth is strong and able to hold it, so I can go back to my life. You know that river in the field? It was all dried out before, but now it's flowing. It's as if we're all alive again."

My eyes teared up a little as she told me what she was seeing and feeling, amazed at the medicine's capacity to bring us out of fear and back into harmony with the Earth.

That was the beginning of a long path for Julie of coming into herself, remembering how to play, and stepping out of self-protection and hiding. She and I still work closely together. She's studying to be a psychedelic guide. It's been beautiful to watch her metamorphosis from that first conversation to now. If you asked me for three words to describe her now, I'd say "playful," "embodied," "wise." She goes to the woods for therapy. She's held in the space where nature and her ancestors co-mingle as one and the spirit seeds are alive and growing inside her.

JOURNAL PROMPTS AND REFLECTIONS

» Consider the most profound experience you've had with nature. What impact did it have? In what way was it healing?

» In an era where we spend a lot of time with technology, do you have any rituals or regular practices in nature? Consider some that you would like to implement as part of your healing journey.

» Write about each of these elements: earth, air, water, and fire. Imagine giving a burden to each of them and how they could help heal the wound.

(26)

Legacy Burdens and Ancestral Relief

Your good life makes your ancestors' lives better.

— Socrates

AS WE MOVE THROUGH THE CLINICAL ARC of the psychedelic heal-ing process, we work at meta-levels. First, we support individuals in the therapeutic space as they move from activated fight-or-flight mode to a more balanced state of repair. To accomplish this, we must meet all the parts within ourselves that have been built as coping mechanisms and pro-tection from the pain of the past.

Coming into alignment with our internal family system pushes us to reconsider our external family of origin and the things we've come to accept as truth. How we think about our family—how we see them and relate to them—stands in need of radical change and newly defined boundaries. As we shift beyond the intellectualized understanding of our family of origin, we begin to allow ourselves to grieve what was lost. In the internal family systems therapeutic model, these embedded limiting beliefs are referred to as "legacy burdens."

There's a lot of dialog in the world of mental health today about "cycle-breakers" and "cycle-breaking." Cycle-breakers are individuals who emerge from an entrenched lineage story of abuse, trauma, or addiction and disrupt the pattern. This capacity to disrupt takes tremendous strength, and requires support and even intervention. It is not easily done with the conscious mind, which is rigidly locked in a trauma response and consumed with management and control. It doesn't have the bandwidth to go into the archives of our ancestry, because it's too busy trying to survive right now. And this is where psychedelic-assisted therapy can help.

Family Affairs

As I've told you before, my father was conceived through an absence of conscious consent when my grandmother was just fifteen. He was born in an old farmhouse with no running water. Poverty inside and out. She had been raped by my grandfather, who was raised in a tradition in which women—especially wives—were property. They did what they were told, and sex was no exception.

When the psilocybin takes me to the dark ancestral cave, I smell moonshine on the walls. I hear her first in a scream and then in a scared, animal whimper. "*Stop,*" she pleads. I sense terror, the kerosene lamp dimly lighting the corridor through which she frantically crawls. The back of his calloused hand with huge, hairy knuckles strikes her cheekbone. Her small five-foot body smacks to the floor. Sometimes she fights back. Sometimes she doesn't. They didn't get divorced, but they didn't live happily ever after. I wonder if any of their eight babies came from love.

Perhaps my dad is the most broken because he was the only child of rape. Perhaps his contempt for his mother and me is bound up in that story of life born out of fear and violence. Perhaps me speaking the shame is an offering to break the curse. He wanted the mother I am, one who *wants* her child. His karma is lost in longing. Perhaps telling our story won't make him angrier; perhaps it will set us both free.

My grandparents' shame became my father's, and his shame became mine. Sexual trauma—passed down the generational line. Like Morse code or an ancient dialect, traveling through time and my family right alongside big lips and sharp tongues. He escaped poverty, but the shame stuck to his bones. No tenderness. No touch. The vulnerability love requires was more than he could muster. He raised me to be hard and gritty, humble and sorry.

When I nearly died of depression, my parents got me help. He didn't believe in therapists, but he paid for one for me because my mother insisted. His only love language was providing for us and working. He was better than his father. That's not nothing, but it wasn't enough. My life looked like privilege and felt like rot. When he couldn't contain his rage, he struck me, knuckles like the ones in the cave.

Time folds in on itself in psychedelic space. Nothing is linear. I am a little girl. I am my grandmother. I'm a teenager. A daughter. A mother. A baby. I see everything at once. The grand, tragic tapestry of my lineage revealed.

I see my sons on the horizon. They're safe. I'm holding back a tsunami of pain so big and old that it feels as if it could destroy me if I let it. But their emancipation from this lineage story is my deliverance and theirs.

The only way for me to heal was necessarily extreme. The truth was too unbearable. My ego wouldn't allow it, wouldn't let me stop running and pretending everything was okay. Twenty years of talk therapy hadn't made a dent. Talking isn't how you repair these kinds of deep, insidious wounds—wounds that are camouflaged into the very construct of my DNA. This work requires metaphysical soul surgery.

If someone had told me I'd grow up to be a mom hallucinating on mushrooms, I'd have said they were crazy. But what we don't heal, we hand to our babies. That was not going to be my offering or their legacy. Years have passed since the emancipation began. The ghosts are gone. The future is wild and bright, punctuated with shadows to help us learn the never-ending dance between purpose and pain.

Now, we ride horses and howl at the moon, and we don't question our worthiness.

Consider your genetics (the hardware of Self) and epigenetics (the software of Self). What strikes you most?
Consider the narratives and belief systems embedded in
your lineage. How would life be different without those
burdens?

Breaking Cycles

The experience described above came from of one of the most challenging
medicine sessions in my healing journey. It illuminated how my personal
trauma was rooted in a pervasive lineage system of dysfunction, mental
illness, and abuse. Understanding this made me both sad and curious—sad
for the loss that went far beyond me, and curious as to why. Why was this
brokenness perpetuating without resolution? How could I make it stop?
This question compelled me to seek answers and work at my healing in a
different way, one not rooted in control, but in a more conscious curiosity—a way that might enable me to eradicate the pain rather than simply
medicate it at the surface.

My intention entering this session had been to understand my father's
pain better. Just minutes into the psychedelic experience, I was pulled into
my inherited legacy burden. Being in that liminal space was hard and
scary, and deeply empowering. From an epigenetic perspective, the experience was essential, because it gave me something concrete to press against.
The figurative cave in which I found myself, viscerally reminiscent of my
father's childhood home, illuminated the point of origin for the pain I'd
carried all my life. It put my story within the context of a larger story. This
made it possible to see myself, not as the problem, but as the potential
solution. This, in turn, made it possible to pivot in my path and alter my
epigenetics. That epigenetic "upgrade" was essential for the quality of my
own life. But even more important, it was essential for my children, so that
the same entrenched limiting beliefs handed to me would not pass to them.

While this psychedelic experience marked a critical change in understanding my self-concept, it was by no means the endgame. The transformation happened in the work that followed, in the ongoing body of integration.

Clients always ask what integration is and how long it will take to be better. The answer to this question is embodied in learning to live within the greater understanding of your lineage system. This takes as long as it takes to tap into empathy. As we saw in chapter 24, true empathy is attained, not by way of a cognitive bypass or a noble idea that we should forgive others, but rather through a metabolization of trauma stored in the body. As we lighten our ancestral load and unburden ourselves, we can begin to expand our consciousness and envision what it means to live as opposed to just surviving.

JOURNAL PROMPTS AND REFLECTIONS

» Consider your maternal/paternal wound. Now consider your mother/father's wounding. How was the way they parented you different from or the same as how they were parented?

» When are you hardest on yourself? What is the fear or belief you hear most resounding in your thoughts? In what way did your mother, father, or grandparents experience a similar fear or belief?

» Imagine yourself as a child—your scariest memory or a time when you felt safe. Was it with your parent(s)? If so, what was the impact of their presence? Imagine/describe how the younger version of yourself might feel better or different if that memory had unfolded in another way.

» If you are a parent or caregiver, imagine how your life might be different had you received the love as a child that you now provide for another.

The Wisdom
of the Wild

Nature is not a place to visit. It is home.

— Gary Snyder

THERE IS NO GOOD EXPLANATION FOR TRAUMA. We can understand where it comes from and how it all got started—and that may be useful up to a point. But there is no epiphany that makes it "all better." How many times have I looked into the tearful eyes of a client who's begging me to explain how the horror of what they endured was even possible? The most honest answer from my maternal heart is to say lovingly: "There is no justification for what is fundamentally wrong."

Healing is not about resolving the irresolvable. Rather, healing lives somewhere on the other side of the pilgrimage for proof, after the ceremony. At the end of a long tunnel and an almost soul-crushing quest, healing waits for us to stop looking for answers and start trusting ourselves. Healing is a vulnerable, brave softening into care rather than a relentless test. It happens at the edge of where our pain meets what remains of hope and we remember we are more than what we endured.

Healing happens in the heart, birthed through the Earth. But what's missing from our lives today is the wisdom of the wild. We've sterilized too much in the name of progress and civilization. If we can remember how to be primal inside the mystery, we'll be well on our way to being better.

There is no completion point in the journey of becoming. There is no erasing of the past, only an open-ended invitation to repair. When we consistently, repeatedly show up to that endeavor, we alchemize pain into something different. It's like watching a wound turn to a scar. The mark remains, but the bleeding stops. What persists is a gut-wrenching, beautiful story to tell. The collection of those stories called forward out of secrets and shame becomes a map to a new life.

Pachamama's Voice

The curandera said: "Your first attachment injury was not being taught to know the Earth as Mother." I felt the Earth move beneath me as she said it, as I sipped the psilocybin tea she had lovingly prepared. Inside this native land, I found an abundance of Mother where there'd been only scarcity before. Discovering Pachamama's voice in the medicine space was like opening a portal to see and hear her everywhere. It required learning a language that had always been humming in the background, only I couldn't discern it before. She gave me permission to be myself and helped me find my voice.

I feel Pachamama rock me every Sunday in the ocean-church where we swim like fish and play like big kids with my little children. I watch her lush vegetation overtake the roads in the springtime when the rains come. I see her great strength reflected in the way water changes the shape of stones over time—slow, steady, and mighty. She helps me remember that I am made of this same might and matter. She shows me the essence of abundance that grows without problems or resistance in the folds of secure attachment, in the lap of her womb. My experience of this great maternal presence is sustenance to my spirit and a salve on my burns of violation. She is milk and honey, and my body is the Promised Land.

Deep inside the mycelium web, I can see, not only the secrets of the past, but the power of shame and cultural conditioning. The culture in which I was raised celebrated the maiden—her prettiness, her complicity, her need to be rescued. She was the prize who could only be enjoyed by others, never by herself. Because she was the symbol of what was desirable, this is what I thought I was supposed to be. Yet nothing about her coyness, her competition, her resignation—none of it fit. She was powerless and, as hard as I once tried to obey the patriarchal orders, my spirit was unwilling to be broken.

The medicine reveals all these maiden wounds and traps as slippery portals to suffering. But in the embrace of Pachamama, something entirely different is happening. I watch the mother and the grandmother, the witches and the crones tending to their work. They are folded into the trees, the forest, the jungle. They blend with the land itself. I watch them weave their way out of the woods like vines, wrapping me in a swaddle under the moon and the stars. "*Descansa*," they whisper in every mother tongue with a kind of reassuring urgency that feels, not scared, but earnest.

Braided into those vines, I finally, completely, surrender the struggle for the first time in my life. It took decades of deconstructing, rearranging, searching, praying, hoping, believing. But I feel held in a way I've never felt before. "You are safe. You are loved. You are protected," they repeat over and over and over, until even my bones and DNA know it is true.

Then I sit up like a baby waking from a nap—content, rested, and restored. There is a huge wooden table in the center of the jungle adorned with flowers. All the mothers and grandmothers, the witches and women of wisdom, sit laughing, crying, holding up the universe with their love and intuition. There is an open chair, and one of them motions to me to come take a seat. "Why don't you join us," she says. "Let us help you. Let us love you. Let us show you what we know."

I sit, humbled and amazed. It seems that, after all my travels and searching, I've found a place that feels like home. Forty years to return to the wisdom of the wild alive inside myself. In stillness, I absorb the energy, the essence, the knowingness of this council of elders. They speak in dialects that my soul recognizes, but that my mind is just beginning to comprehend. They insist that I embrace my witchcraft, my pleasure, my permission to be free.

"Mother must be big," they tell me. "She must know her power and when to wield it. She must understand that her strength is her salvation. Her love is her medicine. No more quiet. No more small. No more sorry."

Each one of them, through their wrinkles and folds, beams a light of beauty that is hard to describe—the pure radiance of unapologetic truth. In the company of these women spirits, I understand that growing older is a journey of mastery and service, not vanity and loss. Reciprocity is my work. Love is my reward. It feels good to be seen and to see.

They offer another cup of tea that looks turquoise and smells of honey and earth. I sip it slowly, knowing there is no longer any rush. No need to strive relentlessly or hurry. I am exactly where I am supposed to be, and I've been making my way here the whole time. The trees in this great forest, this jungle, remind me of the plush, unkempt mountains of my childhood in Tennessee. How far I've come to land in another wild corner of the world.

But it makes sense, the way all great riddles do once you figure them out. The deepest wisdom grows and thrives in the wild where the spirits speak, the animals listen, and repair is always possible. Outside the possessions, the money, the façade—out there in the wild—anything can happen.

I watch as the patterns of sacred geometry and tribal designs color my vision. Vibrant colors of amethyst, turquoise, and gold light up the sky. "Enjoy my artistry," I hear Pachamama say. "My beauty is also my medicine." I feel her move beneath me.

Behind the patterns in the sacred geometry, I see an image of a little boy. I've seen this little boy many times. He shows up in almost every ceremony since I began my healing journey, like a messenger to help me remember what I've forgotten. I can't quite make out his face. It is like peering through a veil. But I see his familiar eyes twinkle in the distance. I feel his consistent energy. He is pure and tender—a little boy of love on a mission to be brave and righteous.

As I think about him, I remember a little boy like this from long ago when I was just a little thing myself. A sweet spot in a mine field of emotional ruptures. I remember him from kindergarten—a little boy who brought me stuffed animals when I was sad, who read books with me in the corner of class. I even remember going to his house once to play, and how magical that day felt. I remember his mother in her apron with warm cookies. Only now the memory feels like déjà vu. I am the mother in this ceremony. But who is the boy?

In the world outside, beyond this sacred space, no one remembers that little boy except me—not my mother or my childhood friends. No one has any idea. "Must have been your imagination," my mom tells me.

Meanwhile, at this big table of elder-mothers in the jungle, they know exactly who that little boy is. "You want me to show you?" one of them asks. I nod my head as she shines a light down the corridor of my house back in the 3-D world of current time. She points the beam of light toward my children's bedroom. I follow the light and watch as the door to my sons' room opens. The light travels up the little ladder of the bunk beds to where my oldest son lays sleeping peacefully. Beside him is little Micah. They are curled up together in the timelessness, like puzzle pieces in a metaverse.

"In my spirit world, logic and time collapse on themselves," Pachamama's voice says. "Let your life be the ceremony. He's your son in this time, your grandfather in the last. How many iterations around the cosmos will you dance? What sacred lessons have your spirits come together to learn?" she asks. "Most important, child, remember that your ancestors are never not with you."

YOUR TURN

Consider your earliest memories of feeling excited and carefree. What was happening in those memories? Who was with you? Where were you? Consider your relationship to logic vs. mystery or magic. How open are you to things you can't explain? How do you think life could be different and maybe better if there were less logic and more mystery?

JOURNAL PROMPTS AND REFLECTIONS

»   Consider the notion of ending and beginning. What needs to end and begin in your journey? How are they connected?

»   How will you practice surrender?

»   If hope is a discipline and belief is a practice, how can you ritualize each of these in your everyday life? With a mantra? An exercise?

»   Explore your relationship with the wild. Where does civilization and structure give way to something more organic and less controlled in your life? What would it feel like to let more of this untamed energy in?

»   What would you need to embrace the wild inside yourself and walk into the great wide wonder?

Conclusion:
Our Journey Ends—
Another Begins

IN THIS VERY MOMENT, as I consider how this book should come to a close, the Earth Mother thrashes in a mighty hurricane outside of what now seem to be very thin walls, providing another perfect metaphor to translate and unpack.

I am tucked in bed with one of my sons on either side. Their gentle breath glides across my shoulders. The rain pelts the windows with a force that sounds like stones banging against the glass. For a minute, like an old habit, I almost panic. What if the glass shatters? What if shards comes splaying into the room where we lie undefended, open-hearted toward the sky.

The thought passes as giant limbs from the neighbor's mango tree fly through the air. I remember again: The Earth is mighty. The Earth is home. I am safe. I am loved. I am protected.

The hurricane reminds me of the Tennessee tornados of my youth, only I am no longer trembling, because now I am securely attached and rooted in myself. I am peaceful. I am home. Healing isn't the absence of fear, but the unwavering presence of love and trust.

A wave of disassociation envelops my body like an elixir of calm. My nervous system has always known what to do and how to take care of me in the face of danger. It's like watching a movie, except this life is real and it is mine.

I enjoy the calm, the steadiness, tucked under the sheet, wrapped inside the chaos of the storm. It's exciting to be this alive. I let my breath get louder and deeper, like a big cat purring. This soothes my children. They stop fidgeting and settle in. They know my strength, my fierceness for their protection. That is my medicine and theirs. As their breath shifts to slumber sounds, the wind and rains begin to settle. It's almost quiet. This is when I hear the Earth Mother loud and clear. She may as well have been in my bedroom.

"The storm was inside you," she says. "Now it's done."

The taste in my mouth is salty and sweet, like freedom and love. The power is out. The air is sticky and humid. Candles flicker in the dark night. My thoughts drift back to what I was working on before the storm began. This book, this story—my story, not my story. This collective saga about how to heal broken hearts. I feel the energy of closure, like the last push before a baby is born. The Earth Mother's presence lingers in the air. The ceremony has found its way to every corner of the everyday. Now life reflects, not control, but curiosity and play alongside an emergence of adult consciousness, budding wisdom.

In the quiet after the storm, I ask the Earth Mother how to write an ending to something that's never truly done. "My storm is labor and deliverance," she says. "Every ending is a new beginning; and every beginning is an end to something else. You've learned to hold trust and you never gave up on love. That is the riddle solved," she says, as the wind brushes like a hand across my cheek.

Giving birth is always a combination of beautiful, hard, and exhausting. It is a great endeavor to pull something from spirit to the Earth without losing anything along the way. It is a quest to bring something sacred from ceremony back as an offering to the land and the ancestors.

I hear the Earth Mother say: "Shhhhhh." She says it many times, until I surrender with all my might. When I wake, the sky is pink and golden. The air is brand new. The sun peeks out from behind the unshakable mountains. Her words are waiting for me upon waking. My logical mind tries to translate the poetic into simple sentences, but she says: "*Stop*. The native tongue is symbol and metaphor. To love a place, we must rekindle the rhythm and the song, the poem and the dance."

Love is a savage beast.
A primal star, pummeling
through the dark
in search of something else
that shines.

I used to be a wild thing in the back
woods, sweaty mountains.
Playing out there on the edges
where fear collides
into arousal,
and it's almost dangerous
to feel this good,
to be so close to the pulse;
so disheveled and untamed.

The colonizers took my body,
and when they did—
they colonized Love itself.
Then it was no longer
a savage beast.
But practical matters and contractual agreements,
taking freedom away
from the hunted and hungry.

But what happens if we go
back to the jungle, and fall
face down in the dirt?
Is it possible to remember
the wild inside?

Orgasm is the Earth's vibration
Hurricanes, earthquakes, tornados—
She's quivering in that place where
pleasure meets pain.
The way you love your children

and it hurts so good
to see them fumble
and understand that is the necessity
of how we learn.

I'm done with
the civilized shit.
I'm ready to be home.
Finally, at last, almost past,
everything built between
my nature and me.
I'm alive again;
native, unafraid, connected,
tuned to the heartbeat of
the wisdom of the wild.

Acknowledgments

So many individuals and groups have contributed to my research into and experience of psychedelic healing that it is impossible to mention them all here. These are just a few of those who have been with me on my journey.

The Psychedelic Somatic Institute in Denver, Colorado, trained me in one of the most powerful healing modalities there is. Dr. Craig Heacock enriched me with countless hours of learning and guidance, and a tranferentially open heart. The music of East Forest accompanied me through countless hours of ceremony. The incredible professors at Belmont University in Nashville, Tennessee, helped open my mind to possibilities I had never considered, while the Buddhist monks of Mainland China and Tibet awakened me to an entirely different way to live.

And above all, I am grateful for the wisdom of the humble indigenous healers, curanderos, and curanderas who have guided my path. *Namaste.*

Endnotes

[1] World Health Organization, "COVID-19 pandemic triggers 25% increase in prevalence of anxiety and depression worldwide," last modified March 2, 2022, *who.int*.

[2] Jillian McKoy, "Depression Rates Tripled and Symptoms Intensified during First Year of COVID," Boston University School of Public Health, October 4, 2021, *bu.edu*.

[3] "About Marriage and Family Therapists," American Association for Marriage and Family Therapy, last accessed November 6, 2023, *aamft.org*.

[4] Rachel Nuwer, "A Psychedelic Drug Passes a Big Test for PTSD Treatment," *New York Times,* last updated November 11, 2021, *nytimes.com*.

[5] Bessel van der Kolk, *The Body Keeps the Score: Brain, Mind, and Body in the Healing of Trauma* (New York: Viking, 2014).

[6] Brené Brown. "Trust in Emergence: Grounded Theory and My Research Process." Appendix to *Daring Greatly,* online in *Research*. Brené Brown Education and Research Group. Last accessed November 1, 2023, *brenebrown.com*.

[7] Ram Dass, *Be Here Now* (New York: Harmony, 1978).

Bibliography

"About Marriage and Family Therapists." American Association for Marriage and Family Therapy. Last accessed November 6, 2023. *aamft.org*.

Brown, Brené. "Brené on Day 2." *Unlocking Us*. Produced by Cadence13 and Brené Brown Education and Research Group. September 2020. *brenebrown.com*.

———. "Trust in Emergence: Grounded Theory and My Research Process." Appendix to *Daring Greatly*, online in *Research*. Brené Brown Education and Research Group. Last accessed November 1, 2023. *brenebrown.com*.

Dass, Ram. *Be Here Now*. New York: Harmony, 1978.

McKoy, Jillian. "Depression Rates Tripled and Symptoms Intensified during First Year of COVID." Boston University School of Public Health. October 4, 2021. *bu.edu*.

Nuwer, Rachel. "A Psychedelic Drug Passes a Big Test for PTSD Treatment." *New York Times*. Last updated November 11, 2021. *nytimes.com*.

van der Kolk, Bessel. *The Body Keeps the Score: Brain, Mind, and Body in the Healing of Trauma*. New York: Viking, 2014.

World Health Organization. "COVID-19 pandemic triggers 25% increase in prevalence of anxiety and depression worldwide." Last updated March 2, 2022. *who.int*.

Index

About the Author

Micah Stover's introduction to psychedelic therapy followed a traumatic pregnancy and birth that unearthed a reservoir of unresolved trauma. The journey to heal those wounds transformed Micah's life. In 2022, Micah began training with the Psychedelic Somatic Institute in Denver, Colorado. She completed the apprenticeship level 1 and 2 certification and is finalizing her certificate of mastery. In Micah's current role as a certified psychedelic somatic therapist, she hosts individual healing retreats and trains psychedelic practitioners. She is committed to education and harm reduction. Micah also teaches an online course called Healing Psychedelics as well as facilitating an experiential mentorship program for practitioners. Her practice reflects a hybrid of study and training from the clinical and indigenous approaches to working with psychedelic medicines. She is passionate about helping others understand the overlapping space where science and spirit meet within the psychedelic experience.

To Our Readers